PRIMARY CARE:
WHERE MEDICINE FAILS

Edited by

Spyros Andreopoulos

Foreword by

Merlin K. DuVal, M.D.

A volume on current health care issues from

The Sun Valley Forum on National Health, Inc.

A WILEY BIOMEDICAL-HEALTH PUBLICATION

JOHN WILEY & SONS

New York • London • Sydney • Toronto

Copyright © 1974, by John Wiley & Sons, Inc.

All rights reserved. Published simultaneously in Canada.

No part of this book may be reproduced by any means, nor transmitted, nor translated into a machine language without the written permission of the publisher.

Library of Congress Cataloging in Publication Data:

Sun Valley Forum on National Health.
    Primary care: where medicine fails.

    Proceedings of the Forum's symposium, held in Sun Valley, Idaho, June 24–30, 1973.
    Includes bibliographical references.
    1. Medical care--United States–Congresses.
2. Medical economics–United States--Congresses.
I. Andreopoulos, Spyros, 1929- ed. II. Title.
[DNLM: 1. Delivery of health care--U. S.--Congresses.
2. Personal health services–U. S.--Congresses. WB50
AAI P9 1973]

RA395.A3S9 1974   362.1'0973   74-9905
ISBN 0-471-02930-0

Printed in the United States of America

10 9 8 7 6 5 4 3 2

CONTENTS

LIST OF FIGURES AND TABLES

Chapter One

FOREWORD • MERLIN K. DUVAL

Anyone who traces man's efforts to improve his lot in the contemporary history of the United States is soon led to this observation: early on, we adopted a sort of "Human Bill of Rights" for our citizens. We have long aspired to a condition in which each of our citizens would have access to food, clothing and shelter, and although we have not achieved fully universal success in our pursuit of this objective, we have continued to make progress. Perhaps, since these commodities are products and America is a product-oriented society, our success in this venture should not be all that surprising. However, we then went a little further and added education as a universal right for all of our citizens. Because this commodity was not a product, its equitable distribution proved quite a bit more difficult. Yet, the rather unique partnership that subsequently evolved in the United States, and was assembled to achieve this objective, knows few counterparts anywhere in the world. Indeed, most Americans are genuinely proud of the degree to which we have succeeded in bringing education into the life of the vast majority of our citizens.

Within the last 15 years, we came to realize that there was little enjoyment in being fed, clothed, housed and educated unless we were also healthy. National surveys repeatedly showed that one of the most important concerns of the average American citizen is the fear that he will not enjoy good health. It was inevitable, probably, that this would give impetus to a movement to consider access to health services as the next most desirable addition to the Human Bill of Rights. Thus it was that, in 1956—during the middle years of the Eisenhower Administration—the White House Conference on Aging enunciated, for the first time, that health care should be considered a basic right for all of our citizens.

Ever since that pronouncement, many organizations and many people have directed their thoughts and their energies to the ways and means by which such a goal might be achieved. But the problems associated with a solution have loomed large. Unlike any other public policy that we have sought to implement in the United States, the problem of the equitable distribution of health services is different because it contains within it a contradiction so basic and so powerful as possibly to preclude its successful resolution.

With some risk of seeming to oversimplify this complex problem, the contradiction can be exposed by examining the essential characteristics of the two elements of the basic equation that are at the base of the contest; that is, the supply and demand elements. Supply is, of course, in the hands of a profession that is essentially self-determining. The medical profession serves as the trustee of the knowledge and skills that constitute its reasons for existence; it selects, examines, and monitors those who would be admitted to its study and its practice, and it accepts responsibility for identifying the new techniques and technologies it will draft into its service. Each member of the profession is a highly trained individual who is both well respected and well compensated. He enjoys the freedom to choose the town or city in which he will live and practice; he selects his own associates, his own hospital, and the organizations with which he will participate as a member. If he chooses to do so he may limit his practice and, at least to some extent, may even select much of his own patient clientele. This adds up to a great deal of freedom for the medical profession. In no small measure it also accounts for the basic strengths of that profession.

The element of demand for health services, however, is less well understood. Indeed, we are not even certain that we know how to distinguish between demand and need. Traditionally, need has been assessed by examining and comparing health indices. Unfortunately, the more one examines health indices the more one learns that they are better expressions of the disparities that exist within a population, with particular regard to economic, cultural, geographic, and life-style factors than they are expressions of differences in medical care. Thus, in the absence of a trustworthy technique for measuring need it was probably inevitable that public policy would come to be shaped, increasingly, by public demand. Since the demand that all citizens should have reasonably equitable access to the entire spectrum of health services at a containable cost arises within the same society that has already given an extraordinary degree of freedom to the medical profession, the contest is thus joined.

How this contradiction is to be resolved is as yet unclear. Within organized medicine there is an increasing body of evidence indicative that medical practitioners are starting to examine, albeit gingerly, the degree to which they may be prepared to accept infringements and encumbrances on their traditional freedoms in order that society's demands be met. Our medical schools and academic health centers also have started to show their willingness to respond to the shifting energies of public policy—a delicate balancing act since they must, at the same time, maintain an appropriately protective stance with respect to their particular academic responsibilities. And to the extent that Congress can be construed as speaking for the public interest recently, it too, has certainly been active.

But the participants in this debate are by no means limited to organized medicine, its professional schools, or the federal government. Foundations, agencies, institutions, organized labor, consumer groups, and others have shown a high level of interest in addressing the problem. One of these is the Sun Valley Forum on National Health. This Forum was established in 1970 for the express purpose of taking such steps as might lead to the improvement of the health of the American people. In three national meetings to date, it has singled out some of the more important issues that must be addressed if an ultimate solution to the problem is to be found. In the summer of 1973, the Sun Valley Forum focused its attention on primary care. Its deliberations and conclusions on this subject constitute the substance of this book. This topic, in the eyes of some, may yet prove to be the most important of all because, in the last analysis, primary care represents the portal of entry into America's health care system for the majority of our citizens; and right now, access is the name of the game.

It is unreasonable either to expect or to hope that all who review the contents of this book will agree with the views of those who have contributed to it. This is unimportant. What is important is that the answer to the question, "What is the patient looking for?" can be found in the book, just as one can also learn, if he did not already know it, that in the last analysis, access is a function of organizational arrangements; it is not a job description. Until such observations as this achieve a more nearly universal acceptance from those who are engaged in this great debate we cannot make real progress toward the implementation of America's newer health goals. This book should help make it possible to take that step.

INTRODUCTION • SPYROS ANDREOPOULOS

American Medicine: Return to Basics?

As a medical writer I have done my share in proposing prescriptions for the ills of the nation's health care delivery system. However, in the absence of a scientific measurement of the quality of medical service, I have grown increasingly skeptical of phrases such as "competent medical care" and the "best medical care" often invoked as panaceas for alleged or real deficiencies.

Unfortunately, the state of the art does not permit medical care priorities to be chosen on a scientific basis. We know far less, for instance, about the availability of services than we would like to know. We have no output measures to evaluate the differences in utilization of health services on levels of health. Comparisons of the American health care system to those of other countries are instructive but not extremely helpful because of social, ethologic and economic differences. Yet, as Fein notes, we cannot be silent because of insufficiency of data. "We can use experience and judgment to arrive at (tentative) conclusions."[1]

This book makes such an attempt. Four professional men and women who have thought a great deal about the American system of personal health services give their opinions of what is wrong with it and what should be done about it. The volume is based on a symposium sponsored by the Sun Valley Forum on National Health, June 24 through 30, 1973. It gives the papers of the four experts who discussed the dimensions of primary care, the question of its accessibility through health education, orientation and practice, its suggested organizational structure, and the impact of funding mechanisms on personal care.

To understand the problems of the health care system, an explanation of the several levels of personal health care is in order. Very roughly, *primary care* can be said to be the range of services traditionally provided by the general practitioner; *secondary care* refers to the cluster of services provided by the

1

specialist and the inpatient part of the local hospital; *tertiary care* refers to the highly specialized services of the larger medical centers, usually connected with a medical school.

The authors make the point that primary care is an all-important contact point between the individual patient and the health care delivery system. Specialists may brandish their skills with flourish, but it is the rare specialist who looks beyond the organ system he is treating to the patient's total needs, both physical and emotional. A return to basics is urgently recommended.

The traditional system of primary care was based on the family practitioner who provided medical attention and advice in significant quantity and in satisfactory time. Unfortunately, not enough physicians today are qualified to fill this role, and there are not enough of them because until recently the organization of the profession discouraged this type of practice. Onerous working conditions, the changing nature of medical education, and the higher rewards and status of specialization all seem to have contributed to the demise of the physician-generalist.

At the symposium it was mentioned that presently primary care has little identity or powerful supporters. It was not explained why, but there is evidence that the absence of a powerful lobby for primary care can be traced to lack of consumer education. McPeak notes that the typical patient today, in his ultimate welfare, has too little influence in the practitioner's office and too much influence in the directions of medical research. In medical care, the patient is the layman, dealing with the expert on the expert's ground, and acting alone. In research, on the other hand, the patient and his family do have a voice. When reinforced by others and further amplified by special disease agencies, by philanthropists, by legislators and government officials, it swells into a vast chorus of dread and fear. The dread of dying from some dramatic disease has produced in our national health effort an imbalance that must be redressed. The cost of the imbalance is substantial enough, but in terms of social and psychological values, and in terms of diverting needed medical talent from primary medical services, is serious indeed.[2]

White states, "We are presently in the position of having a medical establishment educated in a circumscribed setting. A generation of specialists and superspecialists has been led to believe that biomedical research is both necessary and sufficient to meet the needs of all people. We have a population whose anguish with the stresses of industrialized society leads its members to storm emergency rooms, and to seek expensive, superspecialized care for general health problems with large emotional components."[3]

The problem of disparities

There is general agreement that in research and medical technology the United States amazes and leads the world. It has an impressive plant, and many of its practitioners and facilities are outstanding. The total cost of U.S. medical care is now between $80 and $85 billion a year, accounting for about 7.6

percent of the gross national product.[4] But is the U.S. citizen getting a fair shake for his money? The answer is by no means definitive. "Consumers do not believe that the present status of health service is 'optimal' or 'good,' but compared to what?" asks Charles W. Lewis elsewhere in the book. It is generally recognized, however, that for an estimated 75 percent of the population, medical care ranges from superb to acceptable, while for 25 percent, care is inexcusably bad, given in humiliating circumstances, or nonexistent.[5] The breakdown is not simply by social stratum: the rich do not necessarily get the best care, nor the poor the worst. There are disparities in quality and accessibility within regions, states, cities, and between cities and rural communities.

Why can't American medicine live up to its wondrous potential? Here the 31 participants including the four authors agree that the U.S. needs a better system for the delivery of health services. No apparatus exists to define and ensure basic primary care services. But while prescriptions for the ills of the medical care system are easy to make, these experts acknowledge that the complexity of making the needs of future patients compatible with those of health providers is almost overwhelming.

The indirect and basic reason for this problem is that medicine is the only area of the private enterprise system in which the consumer has very little or no control over what he buys. The patient has no way of knowing whether he is getting good advice from his physician, good or reasonably priced medicines from his pharmacist, good technical performance from the subspecialist or the surgeon. The physician, too, suffers from the lack of a rational organization of the medical care system. For the most part dedicated and ingenious, the American physician is overworked and harassed. He is often blamed for the ills of the health care system even though he has cause to complain of the consumer's frequent neglectful habits toward medical care.

Many people, in all social strata, will put off seeking care until their disease is far advanced or incurable. Some, especially among the poor and ill-educated, do not take advantage of care that is available to them. Studies have shown that utilization of medical services is related to distance. As distance increases, the services used—especially preventive ones—tend to decrease. In an example related by Alberta W. Parker elsewhere in the book, the phrase "Ten dollars sick" in the Los Angeles suburb of Watts refers to the fact that getting to the county hospital across town takes hours on the bus. To avoid such a trip requires ten dollars for the taxi. Only when one is really sick is the trip made. A somewhat similar case study shows that in the Bronx in New York City, the infant death rate jumps 100 percent within five miles, going from north to south. The reason is sad but simple. The southeast Bronx is inhabited mainly by poor blacks and Puerto Ricans. Although excellent clinics are open for predelivery and infant care, it takes several hours and several bus fares for a woman to visit one of them, and lacking a babysitter, she probably had to drag her other children with her. The northern Bronx, on the other hand, is largely white, Jewish and health-conscious. There, women go routinely to their private physicians for the same services.

Crisis-oriented medicine

It would appear that because most consumers are "crisis oriented" so are most of their physicians, virtually all hospitals, and most insurance plans. This does not only deny the nation the potential benefits of preventive medicine, it also denies most patients orderly access to the care they need when they need it. Even for the most educated citizen, as Bergen points out, getting such care involves a myriad of obstacles. The patient is first challenged to have the right kind of insurance when he is young and least expected to need it. Then he is challenged to find the right doctor to take care of himself and his family. For none of these are there any reliable consumer guides.

Obviously, it is the physician who should be available to guide the patient through the various levels of health care. That physician should be a primary care physician since many of the most critical shortcomings of the present health care delivery system are connected with his unavailability.

Family care residencies

In his chapter on the organizational structure for primary care, Stanley S. Bergen stresses the sound technical reasons for training more primary care physicians. He notes a trend in medical schools toward development of primary care residencies. As of July, 1973 there were 1,754 family care residencies in U.S. medical schools. There were 145 training programs in operation, 29 more with approval but not yet operating, and about 20 with approval pending. More recently, many prestigious schools including Harvard and Stanford have launched programs to train physicians in primary care medical services. Not only would these physicians be able to care for their patients who are hospitalized with general medical problems, but they would handle the broad range of health maintenance, medical and emotional problems which patients bring to the office.[6] The Coordinating Council on Medical Education of the Association of American Medical Colleges recently issued a report which places heavy emphasis on the need to increase rapidly the number of graduate medical education opportunities in primary care. It concurs that the specialties of medicine and pediatrics should be particularly charged to increase training opportunities, directed toward keeping internists and pediatricians as generalists. Congress has also begun to spell out ideas about how the government should participate in health manpower development.[7] Congressman William Roy (D-Kansas), who was a practicing physician before he went to Washington, believes that students should be heavily subsidized through a loan program during their medical education and be required to provide two years of payback service in designated shortage areas. He also feels that the number of graduate positions should be reduced and the distribution of specialty training opportunities should be controlled by a national advisory group interacting with policy groups in the 10 HEW regions.

While the private physician, practicing alone or in privately organized fee-for-service group practice is expected to remain the basis of primary care for many years, the authors and participants propose a variety of changes for improving the organizational structure of primary care. Prepaid group practice with emphasis on comprehensive health care, health maintenance organizations, and even a greater role of existing hospitals in primary care are among alternatives discussed. However, in the chapter of conclusions and recommendations arrived at by consensus, these proposals are toned down considerably. The experts conclude there is no model of primary care that has demonstrated its superiority and validity to the extent that it should be fostered at the expense of other approaches.

Money and equal access to primary care

Correcting the imbalance between the primary care practitioner and the specialist is a top priority, but it should not be expected to resolve the "equal access" problem to primary care services. Experience with Medicare, reported by Karen Davis, makes it clear that such programs are more likely to favor high income persons, white persons in areas with high concentration of medical services. "If greater equality in the area of medical services is to be achieved, a financial plan should be developed that systematically favors those groups which face barriers to access on other grounds," she writes. Dr. Davis proposes that an income-related national health insurance plan, coupled with direct supply programs and aimed at minority groups and the poor, might be such an approach.

Lewis fears that changes that would improve access to care through educational reforms might decrease the freedom of individual choice, both for providers and consumers of health services. "Whether the society as a whole considers it 'good' to decrease the options available to those seeking to become physicians, and to increase the responsibility of patients through behavior modification or forced alteration of lifestyle may well determine the future pattern of health care in the United States," he writes.

It is mentioned by several authors that medical care, particularly in the hospital, is part a necessity and part a luxury. Whether the American patient, enjoying the world's highest standard of living, will consent to a lessening of demands when he is ill or will actually ask for more services remains to be seen. But that is a social and economic problem rather than a medical issue. The other question remaining is which among the many suggested reforms in this book offer the greatest likelihood of proving practical and effective and at the same time affordable by the nation without substantial inflationary effects?

After more than 10 years of mounting debate, the nation appears to be nearing a point of taking decisive action to remedy the inadequacies of the health care delivery system. The conclusion of this volume, and its main prescription, is that in assessing priorities, the development of improved primary care should be seen as the most important need in the health care delivery system.

REFERENCES

1. Fein, R., On Achieving Access and Equity in Health Care, in Andreopoulos, S. (Ed.), MEDICAL CURE AND MEDICAL CARE, *Milbank Memorial Fund Quarterly*, Vol. L, No. 4, pp. 157-58, October, 1972 (Part 2).

2. McPeak, W. W., The Small, Frantic Voice of the Patient, *Stanford, M.D.*, 9, 1:5-9, Winter, 1970.

3. White, K. L., Health Care Arrangements in the United States: A.D. 1972, in Andreopoulos, S. (Ed.), MEDICAL CURE AND MEDICAL CARE, *Milbank Memorial Fund Quarterly*, Vol. L, No. 4, p. 20, October, 1972 (Part 2).

4. Falk, I. S., Financing for the Reorganization of Medical Care Services and Their Delivery, p. 192, *op. cit.*

5. The Plight of the U.S. Patient, *Time*, February 21, 1969, p. 53.

6. Harvard Acts to Relieve Primary Care Shortage, *Focus*, The Harvard Medical Area Newsletter, February 1, 1974, pp. 1 and 4.

7. Association of American Medical Colleges, *Weekly Report* No. 74-10, March 11, 1974.

ACKNOWLEDGMENTS

I am indebted to the board of directors of the Sun Valley Forum on National Health as well as individual participants for their advice and assistance in the preparation of this volume. I give my personal thanks to Bayless Manning, chairman of the board, and Robert G. Lindee, executive director of the Forum for their support. A special thanks goes to Judy Spates of Sun Valley and Judith Gustafson of New York for the copious help they gave me during the symposium. Most important, on behalf of the Forum, a special acknowledgment goes to the Aetna Life and Casualty Insurance Company, the Health Services and Mental Health Administration of the U.S. Department of Health, Education and Welfare (Contract #HSM 110-73-485), Mary W. Harriman Trust, The Janss Foundation, the Kaiser Foundation Hospitals, and the Milbank Memorial Fund for their financial support of Forum activities.

S.A.

ABOUT THE AUTHORS AND CONTRIBUTORS

Stanley S. Bergen, Jr., M.D. served on the Mayor's Task Force for the Development and Hospitals Corporation of New York City in 1969-70. When the corporation was established to take over the city's $2 billion municipal hospital system, he became its senior vice president for medical and professional affairs. A year later, in July, 1971, he was tapped for the presidency of one of the nation's newest health sciences colleges, the College of Medicine and Dentistry of New Jersey. A graduate of Princeton and Columbia's College of Physicians and Surgeons, he advanced through the academic ranks becoming an associate professor of medicine at the State University of New York's Downstate Medical Center, and in 1968, chief of community medicine at the Brooklyn-Cumberland Medical Center. Earlier this year, Dr. Bergen chaired a special committee appointed by the governor to study the New Jersey Department of Public Health. He is a specialist in internal medicine and the field of human nutrition.

Karen Davis, Ph.D. is a research associate in the Economics Studies Program of The Brookings Institution, Washington, D.C. She received her Ph.D. in economics from Rice University, Houston, Texas, in 1969, where she was awarded the John W. Gardner Award for her doctoral dissertation entitled *A Theory of Economic Behavior in Nonprofit, Private Hospitals.* Subsequently, she taught as an assistant professor of economics at Rice University, until 1970 when she served a year as a Brookings Economic Policy Fellow in the Social Security Administration. She has written extensively on hospital cost inflation, national health insurance, and Medicare and Medicaid. She currently serves as a member of the Health Care Technology Study Section, U.S. Department of Health, Education and Welfare, and as associate editor of the Milbank Memorial Fund Quarterly, Health and Society.

Merlin K. DuVal, M.D. is vice president for health sciences at the University of Arizona and former assistant secretary for health and scientific affairs at the Department of Health, Education and Welfare. A graduate of Cornell University Medical College, Dr. DuVal is considered a leader in medical education. His writings have included such topics as the gap between medicine and the law, health manpower, development of quality standards of health care, rural health, and public health policy. He is currently chairman of the liaison committee of the American Medical Association and the Association of American Medical Colleges.

Charles E. Lewis, M.D. is professor and head of the Division of Ambulatory Medicine at the University of California at Los Angeles. He is a graduate of Harvard Medical School, and also holds M.S. and Sc.D. degrees from the University of Cincinnati. His prior appointments were as professor of social medicine at Harvard, and professor and chairman of preventive medicine at the University of Kansas. He is a member of the Institute of Medicine of the National Academy of Sciences, and has served on a variety of advisory groups and study sections concerned with health services research.

Alberta W. Parker, M.D. is a clinical professor of community health at the University of California School of Public Health at Berkeley. She was graduated from the University of California in San Francisco in 1942, and after four years of postgraduate training in pediatrics, she entered private practice in Berkeley. In 1949 she became director of maternal and child health in the Berkeley City Health Department. In the following 18 years, she held a number of appointments in public health and has taught at the University of California since 1958. Since 1966 she has been active as a consultant in developing urban and rural primary health care systems in the United States and Canada. Presently, she heads a research project studying performance criteria with which to judge primary health care organizations.

Spyros Andreopoulos is a medical writer, information officer of the Stanford University Medical Center and editor of the quarterly magazine *Stanford M.D.* A graduate of Wichita State University and former journalist, he has contributed articles to newspapers and professional journals on medicine, the biological sciences, and scientific communication. He has served on many national advisory groups and study sections concerned with efforts to increase public understanding of science and medicine. Currently, he is a member of a task force of the Association of American Medical Colleges developing a nationwide public information program for medical education. Last year he edited the book, *Medical Cure and Medical Care* (Milbank Memorial Fund). He belongs to the National Association of Science Writers and the American Medical Writers Association.

PARTICIPANTS

Stuart Altman, Ph.D.
Deputy Assistant Secretary for Health Planning and Analysis, U.S. Department of Health, Education and Welfare, Washington, D.C.

James Bax, Ph.D.
Director of Environmental and Community Services for the State of Idaho, Boise, Idaho

Robert Blendon, Ph.D.
Vice President, The Robert Wood Johnson Foundation, Princeton, New Jersey

Carl P. Burke
Secretary, Sun Valley Forum on National Health, Boise, Idaho

Gordon Farquhar
Vice President, Aetna and Casualty Company, Hartford, Connecticut

Melvin Glasser
Director of Social Security, United Automobile Workers Union, Detroit, Michigan

Robert Haggerty, M.D.
Professor and Chairman, Department of Pediatrics, University of Rochester School of Medicine, Rochester, New York

John L. S. Holloman, M.D.
New York, New York

John Iglehart
Writer, *National Journal,* Bethesda, Maryland

Herbert Klarman, Ph.D.
Professor of Economics, Graduate School of Public Administration, New York University, New York

David Lawrence, M.D.
Program Director of MEDEX, Assistant Professor in the Department of Health Services, University of Washington, Seattle

Robert G. Lindee
Vice President, The Henry J. Kaiser Family Foundation, Palo Alto, California

Margaret Mahoney
Vice President, The Robert Wood Johnson Foundation, Princeton, New Jersey

Bayless Manning
President of the Council on Foreign Relations, New York, New York
Chairman of the Board, Sun Valley Forum on National Health

Theodore Marmor, Ph.D.
Associate Professor, School of Social Service Administration, University of Chicago, Chicago, Illinois

Judy Miller
Director, Health Staff Seminar, Washington, D.C.

J. P. Munson, M.D.
Sand Point, Idaho

Matthew Nimetz, Esq.
Simpson, Thatcher and Bartlett, New York, New York; Rapporteur, 1973 Symposium of the Sun Valley Forum on National Health, Inc.

Thomas Piemme, M.D.
Director, Division of General Medicine, George Washington School of Medicine, Washington, D.C.

Nora Piore, Ph.D.
Associate Director, Center for Community Health Systems, Columbia University, New York, New York

Charles Schultze, Ph.D.
Senior Policy Fellow, The Brookings Institution, Washington, D.C.

Henry Simmons, M.D.
Acting Deputy Assistant Secretary for Health, U.S. Department of Health, Education and Welfare, Washington, D.C.

Howard Simons
Managing Editor, *The Washington Post,* Washington, D.C.

Mitchell Spellman, M.D.
Dean, Charles R. Drew Postgraduate Medical School, Los Angeles, California

August Swanson, M.D.
Director, Department of Academic Affairs, Association of American Medical Colleges, Washington, D.C.

Daniel Wagster
Senior Vice President and Regional Manager (S. California), Kaiser Health Plan, and Kaiser Foundation Hospitals, Los Angeles

STAFF

Judith Gustafson, Council on Foreign Relations, New York, New York

Judy Spates, Sun Valley Forum on National Health, Inc., Sun Valley, Idaho

I PRIMARY CARE AND THE CONSUMER

CHAPTER 1 • ALBERTA W. PARKER

The Dimensions of Primary Care: Blueprints for Change

When I attempt to assess objectively the more global problems related to primary health care, my own memories intrude. I vividly recall:

A tired mother waiting with her two young children for long hours on a hard bench in a crowded hallway. An elderly woman with her list of worries who was given no time to ask about them. A businessman concerned about his chest pain who displayed discouragement and resignation when he was told there was a six-week waiting period for an appointment. A fearful elderly couple without transportation, their children long gone, living in a small town with the nearest doctor 18 miles away. A 28-year-old mother who is told she must be hospitalized and has no one to look after her children. The disembodied, bored voice of the answering service in the middle of the night saying the doctor has signed out, and offering no alternatives.

But I don't just remember patients, I also remember many health care providers:

A general practitioner of 58 in a small southern town, recovering from his first coronary and attempting to refuse night calls, yet still swamped with work and acutely aware of the needs of his patients. The pediatrician in a university town finally giving up because of overwork and switching to employment with Kaiser after complaining for years about its presence in his community. The public health nurse trying to find continuous care for her patients. Conscientious practitioners of all political persuasions meeting night after night to try and find a way to offer care for the people in their county without adequate medical and health services. Overworked, overtired men and women, thinking, "How could I do more?" after

15

reading in the morning paper that people in the United States compare poorly in health status with those in Sweden, the Netherlands, or New Zealand—supposedly because the health system is not operating as it should.

Searching, dissatisfied patients; tired, dissatisfied providers—these are the ingredients of primary care for many, and the reason why it is essential to explore this country's needs for primary health care and to consider how these needs can be met in this changing world. Such a task is enormous and complex if we are to move beyond rhetoric into creative problem solving, planning, and leadership.

The health care system, as a whole, displays serious symptoms of disorganization, many of which are most typical of the primary level: unavailable or insufficient services; services widely separated in distance and time; discontinuous, uncoordinated, overlapping, and often duplicated care; unresponsiveness; failure to meet patient expectations. These particular criticisms, if closely examined, are found to apply less to hospitals and medical centers, and more to the primary level situation where people live and die, grow up and grow old, and attempt to cope with an ever more hostile and complex environment. This day-by-day world where people conduct their search for the healer and comforter is the realm of primary care. All societies have created healers to turn to first in time of need—healers who can listen, clarify needs, provide responses, and who will bear the responsibility for the continuity of care. It is, however, exactly in this area of hopeful expectation and anticipated response that dilemmas occur.

My task in this paper is to give some grist for discussion in the form of definitions and facts and to raise questions that must be answered if primary care systems are to better meet the needs of people. David Mechanic tells us that "[t]he particular solutions most appropriate are unclear, and many different types of approaches must be tried. At this point it is more important that we ask the appropriate questions than to settle on any particular answer."[1] I consider this advice sound, and will try to follow it here. In so doing, I shall delineate the dimensions of primary care by first looking at the different operative levels of the personal health care system. I shall then turn to a critique of primary care as it exists today in the United States, assessing the ability of different sources of care to carry out primary care tasks; to the availability of primary physicians and their ability to serve as key providers; and to some key issues related to access and the delivery of comprehensive services. Finally, I shall list some factors that must be considered in plotting a direction for the future.

Throughout, I shall follow some simple but recurring themes, and the questions I raise will be related to them. They are:

- that primary care is more than medical care, and organization and services must accommodate this broader focus.
- that access to primary care is a critical issue and must be recognized as such.

- that adequate primary care services cannot be realized in an organizational vacuum, but will require a structure conducive to change and development.
- that organizations must assume responsibility for groups of people rather than for individuals as has been the case in the past.
- that these same groups must be involved and have a voice in primary care matters.

In exploring these ideas, however, I must in all fairness clarify the vantage point from which I view health care. One naturally starts from the point formed by one's own interests and background. The economist will focus on allocations of resources and how financing will affect services and productivity. The political scientist will look at the dynamics of power created as new primary care organizations are being developed. The sociologist will begin with human beings and study how they interact to build new institutions. The organizational theorists will look at various organizational structures. The medical care researchers will want to know the answers to specific medical care questions. All starting points are legitimate, but all must broaden their focus if they are to be of practical value.

My particular view is conditioned by my background as a pediatrician providing primary care, and my later role as a consultant attempting to bridge the gap between consumer needs and provider response. The strength (and at the same time the greatest weakness) of this particular stance is that it concerns itself primarily with services—the product to be delivered—and secondarily with organizational and financial issues around the production of these services. Nevertheless, this is where I will begin, expecting others elsewhere in this volume to contribute their particular insights in order to complete the analysis.

In probing the issues of primary care systems, I have intentionally been global in approach. So long as this approach is the beginning—not the end; so long as it is anchored firmly in the realities of human beings and their institutions and in the realities of change, I do not consider it a disadvantage. It has been said that by starting with broadly-based questions we free ourselves to stretch our imaginations and open up important avenues that otherwise might remain unexplored. We must always remember, however, that questions, to be useful, must eventually become specific and lead toward practical solutions.

WHAT IS PRIMARY CARE?

I wish to explore the question, "What is primary care?"[2] from several perspectives. First, however, I would like to stress a point that is not often made explicit. Within society many different systems are involved in activities directly affecting the health of people. Highway and city planning, educational and welfare programs, agriculture, control of energy resources—all are inextricably bound to the health and disease status of individuals and groups. Certain organizations and manpower configurations, however, combine to form the *health care system* and are assigned direct responsibility for health and disease care. Within this system, a variety of tasks and responsibilities form subgroupings based on the particular way health problems are addressed. Some concern themselves with planning, some with activities that protect people from unavoidable hazards in their environment, and others with promotive and educational approaches directed to the community as a whole. *Personal health care* is the most visible of these subgroupings. It provides services that help an individual in the context of his family and community keep healthy, get well, or learn to live with a disability. These are the services provided to an individual that specifically concern his *own* health.

Certain subsystems have developed within personal health care that have, to a great extent, operated independently of one another, having different manpower resources, different training institutions, separate facilities, and different patterns of patient referral. Dental care, medical care, mental health services, optometry, and podiatry can be viewed as such variant subsystems. Medical care is certainly the best organized and the most highly developed of these subsystems and it is usually what is meant when the "health system" is discussed.

Personal health care can, in general, be subdivided into three functional levels (Fig. 1): a *primary* level, where the health care system is entered and basic services received and where all health services are mobilized and coordinated; a *secondary* level, represented by ambulatory services of a specialist nature[3] and inpatient services provided in a community hospital-type facility; and the *tertiary* level, which includes the highly complex and sophisticated services available only at a "medical center." This three-level model of *personal health care,* although not a perfect fit in every respect, is nevertheless extremely helpful in conceptually differentiating levels of care and can be applied in situations as divergent as that of an urban ghetto or an isolated and remote Alaskan village. It seems to me that this model works so consistently because the uniqueness of each level is natural, relating to the nature of health conditions, health problems, and disease states to which all mankind is subject.

Effect of Health Conditions on Levels of Care

Let us look at the specific health condition characteristics that predictably lead to these three levels of health care.

1. *Frequency of conditions.* In any particular population certain health problems and disease states will occur commonly, and others will occur very rarely, depending upon the time and place, the age and socioeconomic status of the population, and the environment in which it lives. In addition, unrelated to specific disease states, all groups share in common certain needs for health education, health care for mothers and infants, and attention to personal habits affecting health.

This division into frequent and infrequent health conditions directly affects the need for different levels of care. First of all, primary care can, in the treatment of frequent and recognizable conditions, draw from a small target

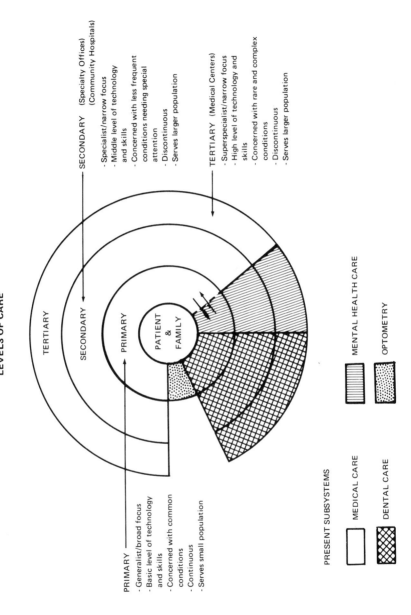

FIGURE 1
PERSONAL HEALTH CARE SYSTEM
LEVELS OF CARE

PRIMARY
- Generalist/broad focus
- Basic level of technology and skills
- Concerned with common conditions
- Continuous
- Serves small population

SECONDARY (Specialty Offices)
        (Community Hospitals)
- Specialist/narrow focus
- Middle level of technology and skills
- Concerned with less frequent conditions needing special attention
- Discontinuous
- Serves larger population

TERTIARY (Medical Centers)
- Superspecialist/narrow focus
- High level of technology and skills
- Concerned with rare and complex conditions
- Discontinuous
- Serves larger population

PRESENT SUBSYSTEMS

MEDICAL CARE

DENTAL CARE

MENTAL HEALTH CARE

OPTOMETRY

population, whereas secondary and tertiary care must relate to progressively larger groups in order to maintain quality. This is due to the nature of some conditions which are seen so infrequently that provider skills and knowledge cannot be easily maintained at a satisfactory level unless large populations are served. For example, the diagnosis and treatment of syphilis is routine for the specialist physician who draws from a large urban area and sees several cases each day; but it may become an exceedingly complex diagnostic and treatment problem for the general practitioner encountering it only at rare intervals.

Second, the frequency of certain health conditions affects the requirements for an adequate base for staffing and utilization of facilities and equipment. A small group of a thousand persons has within it enough upper respiratory illnesses, cases of otitis media, and other common conditions requiring care during any given period of time to produce a utilization pattern that can support a primary practitioner, his staff, and his equipment. A population of millions, on the other hand, is needed to create the demand and use for complex heart surgery teams. Again, an inverse relationship exists between the frequency of conditions and the size of the target populations and this creates natural levels of care (Fig. 2).

Third, the factor of convenience affects the level of health care. Services required to meet frequently occurring health care demands must be located physically close to the consumer. Infrequent conditions, on the other hand,

FIGURE 2*
FREQUENCY OF CONDITION AND SIZE OF TARGET POPULATION
AS RELATED TO LEVEL OF CARE

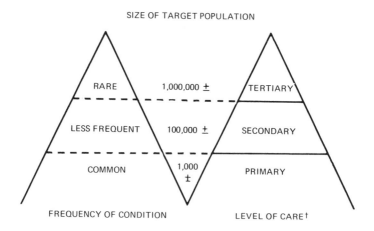

SIZE OF TARGET POPULATION

RARE	1,000,000 ±	TERTIARY
LESS FREQUENT	100,000 ±	SECONDARY
COMMON	1,000 ±	PRIMARY

FREQUENCY OF CONDITION   LEVEL OF CARE†

* Adapted from Fry, J., The Place of General Practice, *International Journal of Health Services, 2* 165-169, May, 1972.

† For the purposes of this paper, I am not considering as part of primary care those services that the patient, his family members or friends provide nor all the services that fall under folk medicine.

requiring services only occasionally or once in a lifetime, do not need to be as close or convenient. Thus, primary care must be physically close and convenient to patients; secondary and tertiary care can be farther removed.

2. *Duration of conditions.* Because so many of the illnesses of mankind are not only common but chronic in nature, there is further justification for locating appropriate primary care sources physically close to patients. The convenience of patients is one consideration. More important is the need to be close in order to collect information about the conditions under which patients and their families live, and to provide continuing coordination of care since chronic conditions require many treatment modalities to which family, work, and economic realities are relevant. Bedside nursing, homemaker services, or transportation may be needed and should be coordinated with ongoing medical care. The coordination of total care, and the gathering of extensive knowledge about the family and community is not so necessary at secondary and tertiary levels, where patients are usually treated for a shorter time.

3. *Acuity of conditions.* Health conditions range between two extremes—those that are slow and insidious in onset (usually chronic in nature) and those that arise suddenly, requiring immediate attention. Acute conditions can be further subdivided into those that need only diagnosis and simple treatment or observation and those that require an immediate referral for quickly initiated, sophisticated, highly technical interventions (e.g., meningococcus meningitis or coronary occlusion). For all conditions with acute onset, care must be easily accessible (physically close and easily identifiable), quickly responsive, and capable of rapid triage and referral to more complex levels. Secondary and tertiary systems, although required to respond quickly, do so only within the limits of the conditions so referred.

4. *Complexity of conditions.* There is a natural correspondence between the complexity of health conditions and the complexity of methods and of resources required to respond. Hence, levels of care reflect a progression of condition complexity—primary care encompassing the most simple approaches; secondary and tertiary care becoming increasingly complex.

5. *Diversity of conditions.* Widely varying physical, psychosocial, and environmental causative factors are at work in many health conditions. Even common conditions, while they may be uncomplicated, are also extremely diverse. Every system of the human body may be involved; every permutation of personal and family relationships can occur. Services must be equally diverse and varied. Assessment of the home, provision of health information, treatment of infectious disease, maternity and infant care, family planning, support and maintenance of long-term illness are only a few of the many services required. Direct help with the problems of living, such as legal referrals or food supplements, may also be needed. To provide or coordinate such diverse services requires providers who can take a broad approach and who can understand widely variable and multidimensional problems. A generalist response, holistic in nature, quite different from that of the specialist, is required. There must be one

level where all the many strands that make up health care can be pulled together. This is primary care.

6. *Conditions requiring an integral relationship with the community.* A large number of health conditions require a close and trusting relationship between the family, the community, and the health care organization to effect appropriate utilization, to collect an adequate and relevant data base about factors influencing the patient's health condition, and to be in a position to help in the alteration of causative and environmental factors. This is particularly true in minority communities where prevailing distrust and hostility of social institutions are common. At the secondary and tertiary levels of care, where the patient is treated on a short-term basis for a specific condition, such an intimate connection with the community is less essential.

Out of these health condition characteristics emerge the following specifications or attributes of the primary care system. It:

- serves a small population.
- is physically close to the community.
- provides a generalized, holistic response.
- is easily identifiable and quickly responsive.
- is able to sort out problems needing referral to the next level of care.
- is continuous in its attention.
- coordinates all facets of care.
- calls for simple approaches.
- is trusted by the community and its people.

The specifications for the secondary and tertiary care levels are in direct contrast. They:

- serve larger client groups.
- may be physically distant from the home and the community.
- provide a specialist response.
- do not need to be so easily identifiable by the client group.
- need not respond quickly to all situations.
- may be noncontinuous.
- are not required to coordinate all facets of care.
- are more complex in approach.
- may be psychologically more distant from the consumer.

In summary, health conditions are different in different populations, and require different provider and system responses. These various responses break down into three different levels of care. The creation of a primary level of care is a natural result of the frequency, character of onset, duration, complexity, and diversity of conditions, and the requisite ties to the community.

Tasks of Primary Care

What should this primary care level actually do? What are the tasks that need to be accomplished? My working definition,[4] which follows closely that of others, is that it must accomplish four tasks:

1. Serve as the entry, screening, and routing (referral) point for the rest of the *personal health care system.* (It is worthwhile to note that primary care, as presently organized, is concerned for the most part with these functions as they relate to *medical* care.)

2. Provide a full range of the basic health care services[5] necessary to preserve health, prevent disease, and care for the common illnesses and disabilities of client populations; and provide the services necessary to ensure utilization.

3. Provide the stabilizing human support needed by patients and their families in times of trouble or crises around health related conditions.

4. Assume responsibility for the continuing management and coordination of *personal health care* services throughout the entire care process (whether the patient is ambulatory or bedridden; whether he is at home or in a community institution such as a hospital or nursing home; whether he is also receiving care from the secondary and tertiary levels; whether services are being provided by the primary care system itself or by auxiliary providers and institutions).

These tasks are, of course, also performed to some extent at other levels. Under certain circumstances, they are expected and traditional elements of secondary and tertiary care. The patient with an advanced malignancy or one having a pacemaker put in place, for example, will require coordination and continuous support while he is receiving services. It is at the primary level, however, where these tasks come together to form a holistic response to patient needs and where ultimate responsibility must remain.

Services of Primary Care

To fulfill the tasks of primary care, an interaction between providers and patients, resulting in services, must occur. (These services, along with a depiction of the derivation of the primary care system, are displayed in Figure 3.) Services necessary for care of groups at the primary level may be categorized as *interventive* or direct care to patients—clinical/technical, supportive, and educative; *enabling,* those that make it possible for patients to receive care—outreach and facilitation; and *formative,* the processes by which the care system is routinized and ordered—entry, triage, and referral and coordination. Let me define each briefly.

Interventive or Direct Services

1. *Clinical/technical interventions (and auxiliary services).* The types of clinical/technical interventions to be used at the primary level depend on the condition under care—i.e., whether it can be handled by medical-dental or allied services, by some kind of psychosocial approach, by environmental change, or by a combination of all three. The process of care, whatever the response, follows similar lines: information must be collected and analyzed, problems defined, plans for intervention made and carried out, and feedback mechanisms

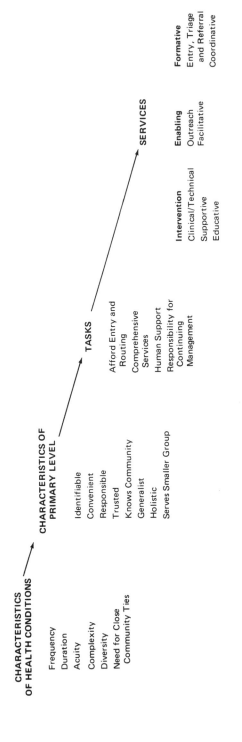

FIGURE 3
DERIVATION OF TASKS AND SERVICES
OF PRIMARY CARE

CHARACTERISTICS
OF HEALTH CONDITIONS

Frequency
Duration
Acuity
Complexity
Diversity
Need for Close
Community Ties

CHARACTERISTICS OF
PRIMARY LEVEL

Identifiable
Convenient
Responsible
Trusted
Knows Community
Generalist
Holistic
Serves Smaller Group

TASKS

Afford Entry and
Routing
Comprehensive
Services
Human Support
Responsibility for
Continuing
Management

SERVICES

Intervention
Clinical/Technical
Supportive
Educative

Enabling
Outreach
Facilitative

Formative
Entry, Triage
and Referral
Coordinative

established to determine progress and failures.[6]

Services may be provided by different providers at different sites and may range from the simple assessment, advice, or temperature-taking provided by a family health worker to the sophisticated diagnostic procedures or therapeutic regimens of the physician. Auxiliary and allied services essential to the primary care process include services needed for obtaining an adequate data base (e.g., laboratory, x ray, developmental assessment), and those necessary in following a treatment program (e.g., pharmaceutical services,[7] physical therapy, or bedside nursing care).

2. *Human support.* Psychosocial problems and psychosomatic responses to life situations constitute a large portion of primary care practice.[8] Their assessment and the therapeutic interventions addressed to their correction are an essential part of the clinical/technical services discussed above. Although given by the same provider at the same time, human support as considered here goes beyond this. It includes emotional and sometimes physical support during times when a person or family can no longer cope with life's exigencies and requires special understanding, comfort, and assistance in weathering the situation.

3. *Patient education.* The disasters caused by the neglect of patient education are so great that I believe it is worthwhile to place education in a distinct category. Health care is of little use if the patient does not reach an appropriate source or if treatment is unrelated to understanding.[9] Only education can lessen this gap by stressing healthful living; ways of gaining access to care; when, and even more important, when *not* to use health care; and by explaining the purposes of different treatment modalities. Although essential at all levels, education is fundamental at the primary level where the focus is on total needs, and where preventive and promotional activities depend almost exclusively on education in order to change behavior.

Enabling Services

1. *Outreach.* In this discussion I am purposely defining "outreach" in a very narrow way. "Outreach workers" in poverty and health center programs have usually been some variant of community or family health worker whose role may include, in addition to "outreach," responsibility for advocacy, facilitation, social work, mental health, and medical and nursing activities.[10] In the sense that I am using it here, outreach refers only to the active reaching out by the health system to the consumer wherever he may be—at home, in school, at work, on the street corner, or in the pool hall. The purpose of outreach is to determine the need for care, to provide information about the availability of services, and to make a bid to enter into a contract (explicit or implied) with the consumer.

"Outreach" is also in a position to serve as an adjudicator of discrepant consumer-provider viewpoints.[11] In this role, "outreach" helps the patient to see his needs as the professional system sees them and at the same time takes into consideration the patient's needs as he sees them (incidentally carrying the patient's viewpoint back to the provider group). This type of "outreach," which may be more necessary in some groups than others, will be discussed in more detail in a later section.

2. *Facilitative.* Depending upon the nature of patient needs and the particular health problems, facilitative services may need to be provided by the primary care system or be so closely coordinated with it that both function as two parts of an integral whole. Services under comprehensive health care programs sponsored by the Office of Economic Opportunity (OEO) and the Department of Health, Education and Welfare (HEW), where groups had special needs because of poverty, have commonly included transportation, translation, babysitting, homemaker services, legal services, and advocacy in relation to social and medical agencies—all services which help the patient gain access to care and utilize it easily.

Many of these should be considered as essential elements of the care process whether or not they are ultimately provided by the care system. Transportation, for example, whether provided by the patient or the system, is always necessary; if a patient is bedridden, someone must always care for him; a mother can never leave small children alone. In most cases the primary care system does not have to consider the solution as its responsibility. To go back to the transportation example, private automobiles or public transportation will in most cases suffice. Yet if fulfilling these needs is always considered a component of the care plan, the health system will be more likely to see that the services are provided when needed.

Formative or Indirect Services

1. *Entry, triage, and referral.* Services grouped around the patient's point of entry to the health system are essential in primary care. They include the assessment of a patient, the decision as to what services are necessary, and the referral to an appropriate source.

2. *Coordination.* Patient care that goes beyond the simplest "episodic" care situation requires some mechanism for coordination. Continuing responsibility for discovering gaps in the data base, avoiding duplication of prescriptions and procedures, discovering contradictory therapies, making sure that therapeutic regimens are implemented, mobilizing auxiliary and facilitative services as needed, ensuring the consideration of pertinent family factors that may influence treatment or outcomes, linking different levels of care—all are part of continuing coordinative management.

A CRITIQUE OF PRIMARY CARE TODAY

Ability of Present Sources of Care
to Carry Out Primary Care Tasks

With this framework of primary care in mind, I will attempt to assess its current status in order to have a foundation on which blueprints for the future can be constructed. The first step in examining the adequacy of primary care is to obtain an overview of the current organizational modes involved in its delivery. Although it is impossible to do this with any degree of precision, estimates are nonetheless valuable for they can provide a general idea of the state of primary care today and the direction in which it may need to move.

Some 840,000,000 nonhospital physician visits were made by the civilian population in the United States in 1969. Of these, 100 million were telephone contacts.[12] An approximation of the face-to-face visits falling into the primary care category is shown in Table I. Clearly, primary care is mainly being delivered by office-based practitioners (Fig. 4). Organized outpatient departments and emergency rooms also play a significant role; prepaid group practices, comprehensive health centers, and free clinics assume a small portion of the total.[13]

There are technical limitations on how the data in Table I were reported and collected. In addition, the figures do not include certain primary care contacts (such as student health centers), nor do they reflect anything about the process and content of care, nor the number of people under care.

Table I also excludes those primary care services performed by other community agencies that lie outside of the primary care system per se. While these services may take place outside of the physician's immediate purview, they still constitute important elements of primary care. For example, entry may be

TABLE I
ESTIMATED PRIMARY PHYSICIAN VISITS
BY SELECTED ORGANIZATIONAL MODES*
UNITED STATES - 1969
(In Millions)

Private Practitioners (a)	442
Hospital Outpatient Departments (b)	61
Emergency Rooms (c)	40
Prepaid Group Practices (d)	21
Neighborhood Health Centers (e)	2
Free Clinics (f)	1
TOTAL	567

* Based on an estimated total of 740 million nonfederal, nonhospital physician visits, excluding 100 million telephone contacts. Assumes that the "specialty" visits of general practitioners, all internists, and all pediatricians correspond in quantity with "primary" visits of specialists.

(a) National Center for Health Statistics, PHYSICIAN VISITS—VOLUME AND INTERVAL SINCE LAST VISIT, UNITED STATES, 1969, Vital and Health Statistics, Series 10, Number 75, Washington, D.C., U.S. Department of Health, Education, and Welfare, July, 1972. (Figure represents office and home visits of all internists, all pediatricians, and general practitioners minus the estimated primary visits to prepaid groups.)

(b) Piore, N., Lewis, D., and Seeliger, J., A STATISTICAL PROFILE OF HOSPITAL OUTPATIENT SERVICES IN THE UNITED STATES, New York, Association for the Aid of Crippled Children, August, 1971. (Figure represents outpatient visits to community hospitals minus 40 million emergency room visits, minus an estimated 25% specialty visits.)

(c) National Center for Health Statistics, HEALTH RESOURCES STATISTICS, HEALTH MANPOWER AND HEALTH FACILITIES, 1971, Rockville, Maryland, Department of Health, Education, and Welfare, 1972.

(d) Estimated on the basis of 7 million members each with 4 visits per year, 3 of which we assign to the primary level using the primary specialty ratio of office practice.

(e) Piore, Nora, et al., op. cit.

(f) National Free Clinic Council.

FIGURE 4
PERCENT DISTRIBUTION OF PRIMARY PHYSICIAN VISITS
BY SELECTED ORGANIZATIONAL MODES
United States - 1969*

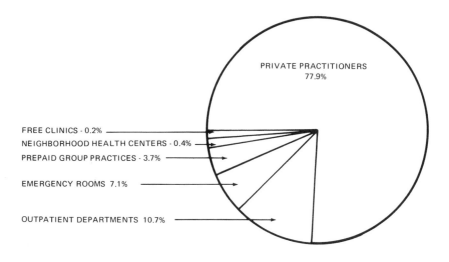

PRIVATE PRACTITIONERS
77.9%

FREE CLINICS - 0.2%
NEIGHBORHOOD HEALTH CENTERS - 0.4%
PREPAID GROUP PRACTICES - 3.7%

EMERGENCY ROOMS 7.1%

OUTPATIENT DEPARTMENTS 10.7%

*Based on figures in Table 1.

initiated through public health nurses or pharmacists, both of whom play important roles in screening and referral. In addition, pharmacists advise and provide over-the-counter therapy and public health nurses perform important educational, promotive, and coordinative activities. Occupational health programs provide entry and also give some immediate and continuing services, as do school health programs and child health conferences. All these services are characterized by their categorical nature, by the limitations in services rendered, and by the fact that few are connected logically or effectively with the receiving systems into which the patient must ultimately go. Although these services are valuable and, if further enhanced, would considerably enlarge the available pool of primary care services, they have tended to contribute to the overall fragmentation of patient care. Their effectiveness is limited by the lack of their integration into a larger system.

The most critical drawback to the information in Table I lies in the fact that, although it provides clues about entry to the system and the number of physician services used, it tells nothing about the other three tasks of primary care, i.e., about the breadth of such services, how much patient support is provided, and the extent to which the responsibility for continuing coordination and management is assumed. Assessing the ability of the different modes to perform the four tasks may not be possible at the present time, however, since the methodologies and assessment techniques required are not yet fully developed. Therefore, in grading performance, I have had to rely on my own experience with primary care systems. This is obviously an extremely crude method. Further it is made more difficult by the fact that organizations, while they may be similar in type, vary widely in the way they operate, and by the fact that individual providers perform differently within any one organization.

In the absence of performance data and with a desire to check my opinions, I surveyed other experienced providers conversant with all types of primary care delivery, asking them to estimate how well and how completely each type performed (Fig. 5). Such a group has had unusual experiences and does not, therefore, represent the average provider's opinion. However, there was remarkably little disparity among them about how each primary care organization performed.

Keeping in mind the limits to such an experiential approach, I would like to briefly discuss the relationship of each organizational mode to the tasks of primary care. It is in this context only that I look at them, disregarding their other successes or failures and the issue of whether or not any one of them represents a model that should be replicated.

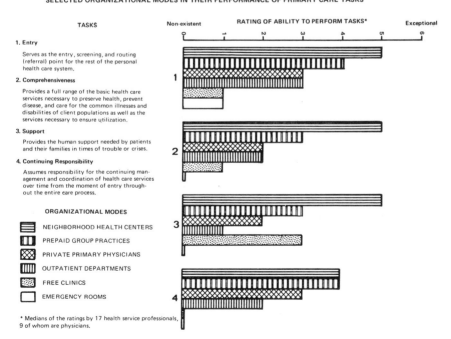

FIGURE 5
RESULTS OF PROVIDER SURVEY RANKING THE ABILITY OF
SELECTED ORGANIZATIONAL MODES IN THEIR PERFORMANCE OF PRIMARY CARE TASKS

Comprehensive Health Care Programs

I refer here not only to the traditional neighborhood health centers developed under OEO and HEW, but also to those rural health programs, children and youth programs, and family health centers that have attempted to broaden the concept of the tasks appropriate at the primary level. Mainly developed in poverty areas, these programs have sought to create convenient, easily recognized, acceptable, and accessible points of entry where triage and referral may be obtained. They have, in most cases, provided a wide range of primary services to their client population with the potential of spanning all the health care subsystems, and they have strongly emphasized the integration of promotive and preventive care with curative medicine and dentistry. They have expanded services to include new ways of organizing communities to attack health problems and hazards, and of gaining the trust and acceptance of the community. Provider teams have tried to support families suffering from the effects of poverty and to act as advocates for them before other social systems. Most important, these programs have accepted continuing responsibility for coordinated family care. The holistic approach of health centers is evidenced in comparison with other organizational modes of primary care.[14] In the provider survey, represented in Figure 5, they were rated at the top in performance of all four primary care tasks.

Prepaid Group Practices

Large prepaid group practices—progenitive health maintenance organizations—come next in breadth of approach. They provide entry to health care that is facilitated by around-the-clock availability and by an enrollment decision made by the patient before receipt of services which allows the program to be clearly identified. Some, as Oakland-Kaiser, have highly developed triage and routing systems.[15]

Services are generally comprehensive in the medical sense. In some instances, generous psychiatric services are included, and a few plans even include dental care. Programs for consumer education, with resource libraries and group educational activities, are being developed. For most patients, however, education still depends on the traditionally limited patient-provider contact. Community organization activities have not been part of prepaid plans; and most prepaid group practices have not developed the "outreach" function to any degree except in the few cases where federal grants have encouraged special attention to be given to disadvantaged groups.[16] Family health workers, public health nurses, or social workers working in a team setting *outside* the ambulatory care facility are not part of the usual provider pattern, although limited home-care benefits are sometimes included.[17] High priority has not been given to the acquisition of information about family and community factors that influence health nor to the follow-up of physician instructions.

Human support for the ill, the anxious, and those chronically disabled or under repeated stress has followed traditional lines—the individual physician, working with social workers and mental health workers *inside* the ambulatory facility. Prepaid groups vary in the emphasis they give to the assignment of a personal/family physician. Most have adopted the pattern of mainstream medicine, with the common provider arrangement being an internist for adults and a pediatrician for children. These providers are not usually formed into a team with shared patients. In many circumstances, patients go directly to specialty care levels. However, coordination exists just by the fact that records can be shared among providers and because there is usually a "one-door" facility in which communication among providers can be facilitated.

Although one might quibble about certain aspects of primary care delivery by prepaid group practice—in particular the lack of attention to accessibility factors, the lack of family orientation, the lack of team configurations for delivery—it must be recognized that they offer an organized form of primary care delivery that has moved a long way toward comprehensiveness, continuous management, and coordination of services.

Private Physicians

Private physicians have been and still are the foundation on which primary care rests. In 1969, visits to office-based, private primary physicians constituted 77.9 percent of all nonfederal, nonhospital primary care visits. Yet, their accessibility is decreasing due to diminishing numbers, limitations on time and practice periods, and their tendency to move away from local neighborhoods into centralized medical facilities. As private physicians increasingly protect themselves by restricting office hours and telephone contacts, people have to delay or turn to substitutes for entry to primary care.

The breadth of services that the private physician can offer is limited to what he and his staff can produce themselves or can mobilize for their patients. Physicians vary widely in this latter respect, some spending a great amount of time and effort in finding services, and others paying little attention to patient needs that fall outside their own office practice. As physicians have become further isolated from their patients, they have lost, in many instances, the facility to obtain important family and community information, and they have lost the opportunity to work closely with the patient in the home setting. Yet, as a group, they have been unable to form close working relationships with public health nurses and other community health workers which would help to fill this gap in care.

In spite of increased separation from the client population, the physician in private practice is still the provider to whom most persons first think of turning during times of anxiety or distress. Even patients enrolled in group plans or registered with health centers are known to leave these sources of care temporarily to seek support and comfort from a private physician. Although decreased availability and time restrictions on physicians, and in some instances their lack of commitment or lack of personal ease, have made support less than adequate in supply, private practice still represents the largest and most important resource for this aspect of primary care.

For all its faults, private practice is still one of the best examples of the assumption of continuing responsibility for patient care management. Riley, Wille, and Haggerty,[18] for example, in their study of general practice in upstate New York, reported that "78 percent of the patients were members of families who were also cared for by the same physician, and 80 percent of the patients were seen on a continuing basis." It is my impression, however, that this sense of responsibility among private practitioners is lessening as patients in the urban setting become more dispersed and less identifiable as a group, as an increasing amount of anonymity is thrust upon the physicians themselves, and as more and more patients use specialists directly without referral. Very often, for example, an internist or a pediatrician may not know that an ear, nose, and throat specialist is also seeing the patient for his "sinus." Clearly, it is more difficult for private physicians to identify the patient group for whom they are responsible and to whom they can remain highly visible and accountable than it was in former years when small towns and cohesive urban communities were the usual practice setting.

Outpatient Departments

Most outpatient departments, although offering entry and clinical services for large numbers of patients, do not score high in ability to fulfill the other tasks of primary care. Usually organized around categorical specialties, the outpatient department provides little continuity and assumes little responsibility for the management of comprehensive family care. Few make attempts to identify patient groups, assign families to a specific provider, or use provider teams. Specific support to persons in time of trouble or crisis is contingent on available clinic time and individual provider initiative. Inadequate data bases, limited services for follow-up and for education, and fragmented subsystems of care all characterize the outpatient department. Many outpatient departments, however, have within them unmobilized resources which could provide patient care for groups in more coordinated and innovative ways.[19]

Free Clinics

During the past five years more than 200 "free clinics" have opened in over 30 states and by late 1972 were providing an estimated two million visits per year.[20] Established to serve alienated youth with special health problems—particularly those caused by drug usage—they soon expanded to include others neglected by the health system. They have been sponsored by women, black communities, and special political groups such as the Black Panthers. From the onset, strict disease-oriented treatment has been eschewed, and the importance of treating the patient as a whole person has been stressed. Innovative human services have been developed such as "hot lines," "calming rooms" for bad drug trips, and "crisis" support for the young person who is ill and far from home.

Free clinics support the ideal of "comprehensive" services; but because of limited financing and staffing, the majority have been able to give only the most basic of primary services, referring to other agencies when more definitive diagnosis or treatment is needed. For the group served, a limited one in most situations, they provide an excellent entry and perhaps the only entry that many of their clients would find palatable. Continuity over time is seriously hampered, however, by the fact that most workers are volunteers and serve for relatively few hours per week.

Emergency Rooms

Emergency rooms, because of their very nature, can be used only for entry and limited diagnosis and treatment. Effective referral is likely only for the most serious conditions. The child with otitis media, for example, may be seen, treated, and referred to the pediatric clinic or the patient's own physician. But this referral is perfunctory and once gone, the child's problem no longer exists as a responsibility of the emergency room. Tasks that the emergency room cannot assume include more extensive commitment to evaluation and treatment, continuous responsibility for care, and human support. The fact that anywhere from one-third to two-thirds of all care in the emergency room is of a nonemergent nature,[21] and that it has become a central source of care for increasing numbers of people,[22] visibly demonstrates the poverty of other sources of primary health care.

Certain insights can be gleaned from this overview of organizational modes. First, those in the lower socioeconomic brackets, except for a million or so cared for by special comprehensive health care programs, are more likely to receive services from organizational modes performing at the inadequate end of the spectrum. Therefore, those with the greatest need for comprehensive, coordinated health services are squeezed into the modes least likely to meet them. Second, comprehensive health services programs and prepaid group practices, because of their organizational settings, are in a position to perform the overall tasks of primary care in a more adequate manner than other types of arrangements. Finally, it is clear that private physicians possess valuable attributes that must not be lost sight of in developing new organizational models.

The ability to carry out primary care tasks, however, cannot be the *only* criterion by which an organizational mode is judged as this criterion does not address other critical aspects of organization and delivery of services. Health centers, for example, may rate high in their capacity to carry out primary care tasks because of the model on which they were patterned. However, for a number of reasons, including the federal guidelines under which they had to emerge and the conditions they faced in rapidly implementing programs in minority or poverty communities, they also possess certain undesirable characteristics. For instance, the eligibility criteria that allowed only those living below the poverty line to be served contributed to the continuance of a two-class system of health care; primary and secondary services were not tied together in a cohesive package; and the grant mechanism of funding, not coupled with an enrolled population, did little to encourage management efficiency or an awareness of patient care costs.

What we should move toward are models possessing the greatest potential for *conceptual breadth of approach* without loss of concern for equity, cost, efficiency, quality, and consumer satisfaction.

Availability—The Primary Physician As Indicator

Availability and accessibility of services, although overlapping phenomena that cannot be considered apart, are not synonymous. "Accessibility," defined as the ability to reach, obtain, or afford entrance to services, is influenced by many factors. "Availability," the actual existence of such services, is only one factor influencing accessibility and is not sufficient unto itself to guarantee effective utilization.

It is impossible to measure "availability" of primary care in absolute terms; seemingly, this could be accomplished with surety only when services stand at zero. In all other cases, "availability" is complicated by locational factors and the number of people to be served.[23] Nevertheless, it is important, when reviewing the status of primary care, to examine what actually exists as best we can. If we are to do so, what shall we count and how shall it be measured? The number of visits to primary care organizations give some evidence about availability (as we have seen in Table I). A count of primary care organizations themselves is less helpful because there are difficulties in clearly delineating the primary care aspects of health organizations and in determining the numbers of persons each might serve.

I shall therefore use the *number of primary physicians* since it is the best obtainable indicator of primary care availability. There is some logic in using the physician as such an indicator since he is the measure on which availability is usually based, and he is and will remain a key and necessary element in the delivery of primary care. "I need a doctor," not "I need health care services," are still the passwords in our society opening that narrow passageway into health care, and the physician is still in almost total control of restricting or enlarging his own and referral services.

There are, however, serious problems in using physicians as the measure. Although of prime importance, a physician cannot *alone* deliver the breadth of services needed in primary care. In focusing on him, we face the hazard of overlooking the need to develop a coordinated team approach to primary care, and of perceiving health care from the physician's limited, although influential perspective. When we look at him as an important indicator of the availability of primary care, let us do so, then, with caution and discretion.

Which of the 194,932 office-based physicians[24] involved in patient care activities can be considered primary or family practitioners? Three groups are commonly included—general practitioners, general pediatricians, and general internists. The latter two, age-band specialists or "specaloids" as designated by Fry,[25] are not totally in primary care as they also spend some of their patient care time as referral specialists, the extent varying with training, interest, and the customs of the area. The calculation is further complicated by the fact that many specialists, such as obstetricians and general surgeons, especially in small towns, provide general primary care. To get around these two overlaps, I am assuming that the secondary care delivered by general pediatricians and general internists will cancel out the primary care delivered by other specialists, and that the three groups *do* serve as a valid indicator of the available pool of primary care physicians.[26]

As indicated in Table II, in 1931 in the United States, the 112,116 general practitioners constituted 83 percent of physicians in private practice. By the end of 1971, their numbers had fallen 55 percent to 49,528, and they represented only 25 percent of those classified as being in office practice.[27] During this period, the population of the United States had increased from 124 million to 204 million, while at the same time the per capita demand for medical services went up.[28] A total of 4,963 general internists and pediatricians existed in 1931;

TABLE II
NUMBER OF PRIMARY PHYSICIANS* AND RATIO PER 100,000 POPULATION
BY PRIMARY PHYSICIAN CATEGORY FOR THE UNITED STATES
1931, 1963, 1971

Physician Category	1931 (a)		1963		1971	
	Number	Ratio (b)	Number	Ratio (b)	Number	Ratio (b)
General Practitioner	112,116	90	68,091	37	49,528	24
General Internist	3,567	3	21,144	11	23,829	12
General Pediatrician	1,396	1	9,255	5	10,742	5
Total	117,079	94	98,490	53	84,099	41
		(1:1060) (c)		(1:1890) (c)		(1:2430) (c)
Population (000)	124,040		186,493		204,254	

* Nonfederal, office-based physicians
(a) 1931 physician figures include only physicians in private practice. For this year, part-time specialists are added in with general practitioners, and the numbers of internists and pediatricians are estimated from the total number of limited specialists in speciality.
(b) Number of physicians per 100,000 population
(c) Population per physician

Sources: Physician figures for 1931 from Surgeon General's Consultant Group on Medical Education, PHYSICIANS FOR A GROWING AMERICA, Washington, D.C., Public Health Service Publication No. 709, U.S. Department of Health, Education and Welfare, October, 1969.
Physician figures for 1963 and 1971 from American Medical Association, DISTRIBUTION OF PHYSICIANS, 1963 and 1971. Part of the decline visible in 1971 is due to a 1968 revision of the series which changed the definition of active physicians.
Population figures from Bureau of the Census, STATISTICAL ABSTRACT OF THE UNITED STATES, 1972, Washington, D.C., U.S. Department of Commerce, 1972 .

by 1971, there were 34,571. Adding these to the number of general practitioners results in a total of 84,099 primary physicians, a ratio of 41/100,000 (1:2430), less than half the 94/100,000 (1:1060) ratio of 1931. Figure 6 (adapted from Fahs) shows this striking decline in the number and ratio of physicians to population for general practitioners and for all primary physicians between 1931 and 1971 in the United States. Figure 6 also demonstrates that the slight increase in age-band specialists in no way compensated for the concomitant decrease in general practitioners.

The decrease in general practitioners is made more serious by the fact that they have customarily seen more patients than the specialists and have worked longer hours.[29] Although comprising only 28 percent of all physicians in office-based practice in 1969,[30] general practitioners were providing 61 percent of all visits, 82 percent of all home visits, and over half of the telephone contacts.[31] Also, they are now older than the average physician,[32] and older physicians tend to see less patients. Thus, serious inroads in primary care resources have been made by the decrease in general practitioners.

To give an idea of the range of ratios of primary physicians to population available in the various states, I have shown in Table III the 11 states with the highest and the 11 with the lowest total physicians in patient care to population ratios, and have then shown how these same states rank in their ratio of *primary* physicians to population (right-hand column). Table III demonstrates that states best endowed with physicians are not consistently the best endowed with primary physicians, and that the disparity between highest and lowest ranking states is less for primary physicians than total physicians.

National and state counts and ratios, while necessary as bases for comparison, tell us nothing about the situation in smaller geographic areas or for particular populations. For example, Robertson's study in Boston,[33] one of the most favored locations for abundance of medical practitioners, showed that between 1940 and 1961 the number of general practitioners declined by 829 or 68 percent accompanied by a negligible increase in internists and pediatricians. Thus, the overall primary physician ratios in Boston dropped from 194.3 primary physicians for every 100,000 persons in 1940, to 175.7 in 1950, and to 96.3 in 1961.

If this overall decline of primary physicians occurred in Boston, what is the situation in less affluent or more isolated areas? Recently a better perspective on the prevalence of underserved areas has been obtained. In order to place members of the National Health Services Corps, the federal government had to identify those parts of the United States where health and related services are not available to substantial portions of the population.[34] So far some 1200 "health scarcity" areas, ranging in size from two census tracts to entire counties, have been identified.[35]

The full impact of decreasing primary physicians is felt when one enters one of these 1200 areas. There were five private physicians for 45,400 persons in a southside ghetto area of Chicago when plans to develop the Mile Square Health

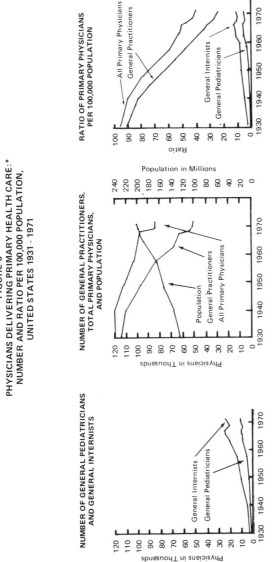
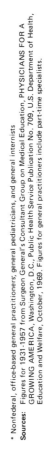

FIGURE 6
PHYSICIANS DELIVERING PRIMARY HEALTH CARE:*
NUMBER AND RATIO PER 100,000 POPULATION,
UNITED STATES 1931 - 1971

NUMBER OF GENERAL PEDIATRICIANS AND GENERAL INTERNISTS

Physicians in Thousands

General Internists
General Pediatricians

1930 1940 1950 1960 1970

NUMBER OF GENERAL PRACTITIONERS, TOTAL PRIMARY PHYSICIANS, AND POPULATION

Physicians in Thousands

Population in Millions

Population
General Practitioners
All Primary Physicians

1930 1940 1950 1960 1970

RATIO OF PRIMARY PHYSICIANS PER 100,000 POPULATION

Ratio

All Primary Physicians
General Practitioners
General Internists
General Pediatricians

1930 1940 1950 1960 1970

* Nonfederal, office-based general practitioners; general pediatricians, and general internists

Sources: Figures for 1931-1957 from Surgeon General's Consultant Group on Medical Education, PHYSICIANS FOR A GROWING AMERICA, Washington, D.C., Public Health Service Publication No. 709, U.S. Department of Health, Education and Welfare, October, 1969. Figures for general practitioners include part-time specialists.

Figures for 1963-1971 from American Medical Association, DISTRIBUTION OF PHYSICIANS IN THE UNITED STATES, 1963 THROUGH 1971. Part of the decline visible in 1968 is due to a revision of the series that year which changed the definition of active physicians.

Population figures from Bureau of the Census, STATISTICAL ABSTRACT OF THE UNITED STATES, 1972, Washington, D.C., U.S. Department of Commerce, 1972.

TABLE III
COMPARISON OF RANK ORDER OF STATES BY RATIO OF PHYSICIANS TO POPULATION FOR TOTAL PHYSICIANS (A) AND FOR PRIMARY HEALTH CARE PHYSICIANS (B) UNITED STATES, 1971

	State (a)	(A) Total Physicians*			(B) Primary Health Care Physicians**					
		Number	Ratio (b)	Rank Order	General Practitioners	Internists	Pediatricians	Total Number	Ratio (b)	Rank Order
	D.C.	2,501	344	1	165	269	76	510	70.2	1
	New York	36,370	198	2	4,409	3,530	1,466	9,405	51.2	3
	Mass.	9,825	171	3	1,281	906	381	2,568	44.8	12
	California	33,010	166	4	6,388	3,376	1,422	11,186	56.3	2
Eleven Highest Ratio States	Conn.	4,985	163	5	588	547	245	1,380	45.0	11
	Maryland	6,167	157	6	720	556	255	1,531	38.9	25
	Colorado	3,318	148	7	575	296	173	1,044	46.6	8
	Vermont	666	145	8	129	75	28	232	50.7	4
	R.I.	1,318	142	9	183	136	71	390	42.1	17
	Hawaii	1,009	137	10	182	105	76	363	49.2	5
	Penn.	15,646	132	11	3,029	1,241	518	4,788	40.4	20
	Indiana	4,738	90	41	1,518	312	156	1,986	37.7	31
	Wyoming	301	89	42	120	23	6	149	44.2	15
	Oklahoma	2,277	88	43	575	197	91	863	33.5	44
	Idaho	625	86	44	248	49	28	325	44.6	14
Eleven Lowest Ratio States	N. Dakota	521	85	45	171	49	20	240	39.2	23
	S. Carolina	2,160	85	46	620	149	96	865	33.9	43
	Arkansas	1,589	82	47	556	111	49	716	37.0	34
	Alabama	2,747	80	48	680	227	136	1,043	30.2	51
	Alaska	214	75	49	72	20	15	107	37.5	32
	Miss.	1,652	75	50	539	106	77	722	32.7	47
	S. Dakota	484	73	51	187	35	19	241	36.4	37
Total U.S.		261,335	128	—	49,528	23,829	10,742	84,099	41.2	—

(a) 50 states plus Washington, D.C. included
(b) Number of physicians per 100,000 population
 * Nonfederal physicians in patient care
** Nonfederal, office-based general practitioners, general internists, general pediatricians

Source: American Medical Association, DISTRIBUTION OF PHYSICIANS IN THE UNITED STATES — 1971, Chicago, 1972.

Center were initiated.[36] In the area of the Bronx now served by the Martin Luther King, Jr. Health Center, there were some three private physicians for 50,000 persons.[37] Rural areas face equally severe deprivation in this respect. Many rural counties and small towns have no physician, and vigorous recruiting efforts have ended in failure.[38]

One example of rural deprivation is the situation that existed in the four Arkansas counties around Pine Bluff (Fig. 7). In Jefferson County, the market center of the area, 88,187 people were served by 26 primary physicians in 1969, a ratio of 29 primary physicians/100,000 (1:3392). In Cleveland and Lincoln Counties, where great distances are involved in traveling to health care, and

FIGURE 7
RATIO OF PRIMARY PHYSICIANS PER 100,000 POPULATION
FOUR COUNTIES IN ARKANSAS - 1969

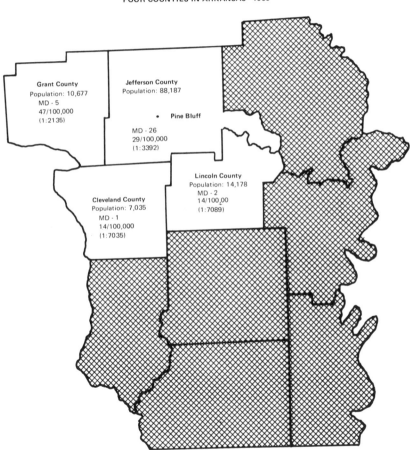

Source: Jefferson County - Pine Bluff Health Center, Comprehensive Health Services Application, Pine Bluff, May 1, 1970.

where large numbers of persons live in poverty with few financial or transportation resources, three primary physicians served 21,213 people, a ratio of 14/100,000 (1:7071).[39] Certainly a catastrophic situation from any view, but one that has more significance when the poverty, the high prevalence of illness among lower socioeconomic groups, and the lack of organized efforts to provide services are taken into account.

The Pine Bluff example makes it quite clear that overall numbers and ratios are not sufficient in assessing availability. It is also important to determine how providers are distributed and how easily they can be reached by those that need them. Maldistribution is a serious problem that compounds the quantitative deficiency of primary physicians.

But what is the optimal number of primary physicians and how can their number be estimated? It is mandatory in this regard that the *health care needs* of the group in question be documented and analyzed first and then the skills and service required to meet them projected. Only through this process can an allocation of tasks among primary providers be made and the number and *type* of provider most appropriate for the circumstances determined.[40]

Schonfeld, Heston, and Falk,[41] using methods first developed for the Lee-Jones report of 1933,[42] have projected the need for primary care physicians in the United States. They based their projections on professional opinions about the services needed to provide good medical care (where pediatricians and internists provide for all personal health needs except those relating to dental, mental, and obstetrical problems, and adult routine physicals), and on estimates of the incidence and prevalence of health conditions requiring care. They made estimates of the number of primary physicians needed to care for acute conditions, for chronic conditions, and for newborn and well-child care, and added these estimates together to arrive at a figure of 133 primary physicians per 100,000 (1:750). For the population of the United States, therefore, 266,000 primary physicians would be needed, in contrast to the 120,000 (59/100,000) that they calculated were actually available in 1970.[43]

Two caveats must be added about this approach and its results. First, calculations may be skewed by the fact that projections about the services needed were based on the opinions of medical specialists. Second, the projections do not address the central issue of who can best carry out such primary care services—physicians, others, or some combination—but instead are based on the assumption that internists and pediatricians perform traditional medical care tasks without delegation.

If primary physicians were placed in different organizational settings with staffing patterns and task assignments altered, other ratios could emerge. The delivery structure is of overriding importance in this regard. It is interesting to examine the prepaid group practices, where relatively precise measures of physicians to population ratios are available and where the arrangement and relative number of specialists to primary physicians is without a doubt one of the factors influencing primary physician rates[44, 45] (Table IV).

TABLE IV
NUMBER OF PHYSICIANS AND SUPPORT SPECIALISTS AND RATIO TO MEMBERSHIP - 1970
SELECTED PREPAID GROUP PLANS

	HIP	Kaiser Oakland	Kaiser Los Angeles	Kaiser Portland	Group Health Puget Sound	Group Health Assoc., D.C.	Harvard Community Health Plan
MEMBERSHIP (000)	780	962	900	145	136	75.5	36
PRIMARY PHYSICIANS							
Family Practitioners	116	114	391 (a)	-	40	-	-
Internists	190	297		34	18	34	18
Pediatricians	172	158	138	14	15	15	
TOTAL PRIMARY	478	569	529	48	73	49	18
% OF ALL PHYSICIANS	64%	57%	59%	48%	57%	73%	52%
RATIO OF PRIMARY PHYSICIANS TO MEMBERSHIP	61 per 100,000 (1:1630)	59 per 100,000 (1:1690)	59 per 100,000 (1:1700)	33 per 100,000 (1:3020)	54 per 100,000 (1:1860)	65 per 100,000 (1:1540)	50 per 100,000 (1:2000)
SPECIALTY SUPPORT							(b)
Obs./Gyn.	86	92	100	10	14	7	
General Surgeons	47	72	90	18	8	8	
Orthopedists	31	44	26	5	5	-	
Radiologists	31	35	27	3	4	2	
Ophthalmologists	23	30	20	3	3	-	
Otolaryngologists	16	23	20	3	4	-	
Psychiatrists	16	20	-	1	-	-	3.6
Urologists	8	14	20	3	3	-	
Dermatologists	8	28	20	-	4	-	
Plastic Surgeons	-	2	-	-	-	-	
Neurologists	-	7	10	-	-	-	
Neurosurgeons	-	7	-	1	2	-	
Anesthesiologists	-	31	10	4	4	-	
Pathologists	-	15	10	1	3	1	
Physiatrists	-	8	10	-	-	-	
TOTAL SPECIALISTS	266	428	363	52	54	18	16.4
RATIO OF SPECIALTY SUPPORT TO MEMBERSHIP	34 per 100,000 (1:2930)	44 per 100,000 (1:2250)	40 per 100,000 (1:2480)	36 per 100,000 (1:2800)	40 per 100,000 (1:2520)	24 per 100,000 (1:4190)	45 per 100,000 (1:2200)
TOTAL NUMBER OF PHYSICIANS	744	997	892	100	127	67	34.4
RATIO OF TOTAL PHYSICIANS TO MEMBERSHIP	95 per 100,000 (1:1050)	104 per 100,000 (1:970)	99 per 100,000 (1:1010)	69 per 100,000 (1:1450)	93 per 100,000 (1:1070)	89 per 100,000 (1:1130)	96 per 100,000 (1:1050)

(a) Internists included in count of family practitioners.
(b) All individual specialty support figures not available.

Sources: Figures for all plans except the Harvard Community Health Plan are for 1970 and were computed from Mason, H., Manpower Needs by Specialty, *Journal of the American Medical Association*, 219, 1621-1626, March 20, 1972.

Figures for Harvard Community Health Plan are for 1973 as per Dorsey, J., Personal Communication, June, 1973.

The use of mid-level practitioners in prepaid plans, now becoming increasingly common, but about which precise documentation is not yet available, is also bound to have profound effects on primary physician ratios. The Columbia Plan, for example, which assumes that physicians will work in a well-organized team structure with "health associates" and family health workers, is projecting a ratio of 20/100,000 or one primary physician per 5000 enrollees.[46] This is a marked contrast to the present 50/100,000 primary physician ratio at Harvard Community Health Plan,[47] the 1970 ratios at Oakland and Los Angeles Kaiser (59/100,000), Health Insurance Plan of Greater New York (61/100,000), and Group Health Association of Washington, D.C. (65/100,000).[48]

Using 1970 population figures, if the Harvard Plan ratios were projected for the country as a whole, 100,000 primary physicians would be required in the United States. If the Kaiser-Los Angeles ratios were used, the projection would be 120,000, a far cry from the 266,000 projected by Schonfeld, but identical to his estimate of 120,000 primary physicians available in 1970. If in fact the 1:5000 ratio of the Columbia Plan should ever prove feasible, and if distribution problems were solvable, only 40,000 primary physicians could serve the population of the United States.

What can we say, in summary, about availability of primary physicians as key providers of primary care?

1. The number of primary physicians to population is decreasing.
2. As presently organized and distributed, the available primary physicians are not able to meet the primary care needs of the nation.
3. Optimal rates for physicians to population are dependent not only on the needs of the population, but also on the patterns of specialist usage, substitution of other providers, and task assignment within primary health care teams. Evidence suggests that if tasks were reassigned in a more rational manner, and a more even distribution could be assured, massive increases in primary care physicians would be unnecessary.

Current Strategies to Increase the Availability of Primary Care Providers

Fahs and Peterson[49] have projected the demise of general practice by 2000 A.D. (Fig. 8). This threat of the loss of general practitioners is not reflected in a decrease in emphasis on primary care; just the opposite is happening. The squeeze between provider time and patient demand and the increasing unavailability of providers in rural and urban ghetto areas have not gone unnoticed by providers and consumers. At the same time, the level of consumer sophistication about health and health care, and the importance of efficiency factors have risen. The question of how to replace the services of the general practitioner and make them appropriate to present day needs has become a focal point of national concern.

As previously shown in Table I, the majority of people now obtain primary care from private physicians. Certain factors related to private practice,

FIGURE 8
RECENT CHANGES IN NUMBERS AND RATIO OF GENERAL PRACTITIONERS
PER 100,000 POPULATION, WITH FUTURE PROJECTIONS*

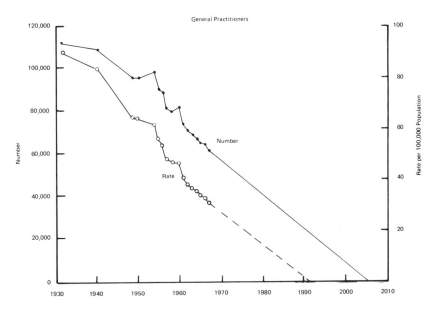

*Reproduced from Fahs, I.J. and Peterson, O.L., The Decline of General
Practice, *Public Health Reports*, 83, 267-270, April, 1968.

however, must be taken into account as one reviews strategies to overcome the
unavailability of primary care providers: 1) private fee-for-service practice—solo
or small group—has so many constraints placed upon it that in its present form it
cannot be expected to serve as the main source of primary care in the future if
comprehensiveness, effective task delegation, and equity are to be realized; 2)
the greatest block to private practice becoming a successful and effective mode
lies in its lack of organizational structure around which manpower and services
can be developed and arranged; and 3) the advantages of autonomy and private
entrepreneurship in private primary practice are becoming less attractive as its
disadvantages mount. Therefore, it is fast losing its ability to attract and hold
physicians.

What are some of the current strategies to increase the availability of
primary care providers?

1. *The production of primary physicians.* One of the most prominent strategies to overcome shortages in personal health care has been to increase the *overall production of physicians.* I would suggest, however, that rather than a "physician shortage," we are facing an imbalance between the primary care provider and the specialist, and an increasingly noticeable geographic maldistribution of primary physicians. New medical schools and increased class sizes that produce more physicians will not guarantee more primary care providers nor a change in location where they will ultimately practice. If emerging physicians are to be more concerned with primary care than those of the past, there must be changes in the way students are selected, in the process of medical education, in the characteristics of those seen as academic leaders, in the academic emphasis on research, and in the relationship of the medical school to the community.

Postgraduate training closely attuned to the health problems seen in primary practice and "specialized" status are being used to create a new body of *family practitioners* who will hopefully find general practice more satisfying and higher in prestige than did their predecessors.[50] Whether this will attract and hold young men and women in the present practice environment is yet to be seen. I predict it will not. Medical education will, and must, continue to emphasize high quality performance in scientific and technological areas, and physicians trained in this way are not likely to be content with being the sole providers of primary care services in the future. Family practice is a rational response to the problem of delivering primary care. But if physicians have to practice without access to accepted skills and equipment, to work in isolation in rural areas or the inner city, to carry the burden of practice without a team effort, it may not prove to be a viable solution. Organizational structures may be necessary to nurture and protect it.

If one looks to the *pediatrician-internist dyad* either to replace or to continue to supplement the primary generalist, similar constraints will be encountered. At their present rate of production, such specialists cannot be expected to replace the generalist entirely. In addition, the move out of primary practice into subspecialties is increasing. The pediatrician, in particular, is becoming dissatisfied with his workload, the scope of his services, and his reimbursement. If not given more extensive organizational support, such specialists may also find private, unstructured, primary practice less than attractive, particularly in underserved areas.

2. *Use of mid-level practitioners.* A swiftly accelerating and somewhat astounding development is the creation and acceptance of mid-level practitioners—physician assistants and nurse practitioners. Many, of course, are being trained for specialty practice, but others are planned as generalists for the primary health care team.[51] Although the use of such mid-level workers can certainly affect individual physician productivity, it may have little overall effect on improving distribution or availability of primary care services if it stays tied to fee-for-service private practice and to physicians as presently distributed.

The extent of "substitutability" of physicians by mid-level practitioners is as yet unknown. In remote areas, such workers, under supervision, are now successfully assuming almost the entire primary care load. In urban America what will eventually emerge will depend on the organizational setting and on the urgency of the need to substitute. Certainly if integrated into a cohesive team approach, mid-level workers may have profound effects on primary care.[52]

3. *Redistribution of primary care providers.* Certain strategies specifically address the problem of redistribution of primary care providers. One method is the *loan forgiveness* program of many states which allows a student to repay his loan by serving a number of years in a scarcity area. So far these programs have had little success in accomplishing a redistribution of primary physicians. This is also the case with other incentives in the form of provision of offices or practice subsidization.[53]

Preferential selection of new types of students, especially those from minority and ghetto areas, has been tried, not only to redress old discriminatory patterns, but to redistribute health manpower. It has also been suggested that those with rural backgrounds be preferentially admitted to medical schools to swell the family practice ranks for rural America, since physicians with such backgrounds have been more likely to go back into practice in rural areas.[54] Whether such factors will continue to be operative around rurality is open to question. In any case, the results of these selective mechanisms will not be known for many years.

The Area Health Education Centers have, as one of their main objectives, the redistribution of primary care providers. To this end, emphasis is being placed on building "intellectual oases" and unique *primary care residency programs* in underserved areas, since it is known that physician location has been strongly influenced by the site of residency.[55]

The *National Health Service Corps* program is also attempting to redistribute professionals by placing them for short assignments in underserved areas. It is hoped that these young professionals will put down roots and remain.[56] However, no attempt is being made to change the organizational structure into which these young women and men go. They must, therefore, adapt to some of the worst aspects of primary care as practiced in "health care scarcity" areas—a situation certainly offering little inducement to remain. While this program may be successful in individual instances, my limited contact suggests that it may fail to have a significant impact on distribution, especially in view of the ending of the draft.

Other countries, facing similar situations in which highly trained physicians and nurses do not wish to spend their lives in areas with inadequate practice environments and with few personal amenities, have passed *draft laws* requiring graduates of professional schools to serve temporarily in scarcity areas. Hopefully, this will not be necessary in the United States but the possibility exists, that if other measures do not work, it will be tried.

The *neighborhood health centers* represent a massive effort to overcome maldistribution. Placed in underserved areas, they have had to recruit large numbers of health professionals for localities where few existed prior to funding, a task that has not proven to be as difficult as many anticipated. Although salaries have been high, the success in recruitment has probably been related more to the excitement of being involved in a new, highly publicized endeavor—seen by many as an important step forward in health care delivery—than to personal financial advantage. Whether or not these professionals will remain and become integral and lasting members of the community is as yet unknown. So far, worries about the instability of funding, the often horrendous effects of community politics, the fear of loss of professional autonomy, and the traumas associated with new organizational development have all mitigated against their retention. The little evidence I have would suggest that health centers cannot, at this stage of their development, hope to emulate in any manner the low turnover rate of the well-organized prepaid health plans.[57]

It seems unlikely that maldistribution will be overcome without organizational change within primary care systems so that they will be in a position to recruit health professionals, maintain their allegiance, create acceptable professional environments, provide adequate financial rewards and fringe benefits and, most important, provide an atmosphere in which the physician obtains personal satisfaction.[58] The ability to develop manpower arrangements that can extend services into seriously depressed scarcity areas can only be accomplished through such a systematic approach.

4. *Unplanned developments.* Other activities to overcome inadequacies of primary care, unplanned in nature, are becoming evident. Chiropractors have become the primary care providers in some rural communities lacking sufficient physician strength.[59] Among the young, self-help health collectives are on the rise. In this latter case, it is not only the numerical shortage which acts as the trigger mechanism; traditional medical care is seen as inappropriate and insensitive, provided in male chauvinistically controlled organizations by professionals allowing little questioning of professional prerogatives and little freedom for patients to acquire knowledge or control over their own bodies, and having too little emphasis on health in contrast to disease. The movement away from traditional providers and traditional institutions by the young will prove to be, I am convinced, an important one in the history of American health care; it is already changing provider attitudes.

Accessibility of Primary Care

Availability of primary care services is naturally a first requirement for their use. But the ability of individuals to get to care is just as essential. Many interrelated factors may intervene between the services available and the people in need of them. The following analogy conveys the multifaceted nature of access:

A building lies in a valley. Most people in the area want to reach the building, but it is surrounded by a high wall. In the wall are many closed doors. Some people have keys and can get easily through the doors. For others, there is no way to get in except to climb over the wall. Whether or not they can do this depends on many factors—the height of the wall, how easy it is to scale, or whether spikes are placed at the top. It also will depend on the person climbing—his strength and agility, his sense of urgency, and his belief that he can do it and that the effort will be worthwhile.

Primary care systems, if they are to ensure equity of health care services, must identify their consumer groups and, within each, those people blocked from care or forced to expend proportionately larger amounts of money, time, and effort than others in order to utilize it. Once these groups have been identified, the factors barring entrance to the primary care system, or making entrance difficult, must be determined and strategies devised for their elimination or amelioration.

There are basically three different ways to identify access factors: 1) self assessment by providers, 2) gathering information from consumers themselves, and 3) evaluative studies. Each of these methods are discussed in more detail below. The value of each will vary according to the size of the population served and the complexity of the particular factors limiting access. Surveys and elaborate studies may not be needed at all in many cases. We already know that the poor of Beaufort-Jasper County, South Carolina, living in outlying hamlets around old plantation sites with no autos and little cash, will need transportation service to get to health care. We do not need to prove that people living in the remote San Luis Valley of Colorado, descendants of early settlers and who speak only Spanish, need translators if they are to take advantage of the services of English-speaking physicians and nurses.

The body of knowledge obtained from general research on utilization behavior may also be of assistance in determining what limits access in operational settings. It can lend an overall understanding of the many factors—socioeconomic, cultural, and behavioral—that together influence how health care is used. But research findings applicable to one setting cannot tell a primary care program what keeps its particular clients from using care. This must be ascertained specifically for the population served.

1. *Self-assessment by providers.* It is often forgotten that, in addition to the physician, each worker in a health program also has information and insights that may be of inestimable value. Receptionists, secretaries, telephone operators, medical aides, transportation workers, and nurses can all assist in the accumulation of evidence, not only about outside factors that prevent patients from obtaining care, but, more important, about the characteristics of the organization itself that block usage.

2. *Information from consumers.* Provider groups seldom survey their patients to identify what blocks them from care and even less often do they survey the nonutilizing population. (Obviously, a system that cannot identify its

total consumer group is in no position to identify nonutilizers.) Although such studies always present problems of interpretation, they can be very useful. For example, a recent study of the members of a carpenters' union belonging to Kaiser[60] showed that problems such as long waiting and lack of personal physicians were causing consumers to turn to providers outside the system. A Watts Health Center survey[61] uncovered a number of factors that limited access to care such as long waiting, manner of treatment by the staff, distance from home, and lack of awareness of center services.

Although surveys provide quantifiable information, certain other kinds of information from consumers can only be obtained through personal encounters between consumers and system planners. To me, one of the most rewarding aspects of working closely with consumer groups has been to be directly and forcibly presented with the facts of utilization as seen from the consumer's viewpoint. For example, I was told by a black consumer group in one small town in the South that physicians having two waiting rooms were not used to the same extent as those who had only one. A black woman, active in civil rights groups, told me of her fear of going to physicians in her particular community because she thought they would take revenge on her through choice of medical treatment. In many situations I have noted that resentment of what is seen as physician insensitivity and discriminatory practice actually keeps people from obtaining health care services.

3. *Evaluative studies.* A "before and after" evaluation of measures such as utilization, patterns of utilization, or patient satisfaction during a period when one factor bearing on access has been altered, is one of the best, although seldom obtainable, ways to pinpoint specific accessibility factors. If the addition of transportation to a system, or the placement of a satellite clinic in the neighborhood, or the development of a new cadre of family health workers is followed by a change in the way consumers use services, we begin to have evidence of influences on accessibility.

In a Rochester, New York study,[62] for example, the introduction of the Title XIX program was shown to increase the number of patients who turned to the emergency room for care—accessibility to private physicians actually being decreased, probably because of physician refusal to accept Medicaid patients. Also in Rochester, when a neighborhood health center was placed in one area, it markedly decreased emergency room use for those in its catchment area, whereas a control group in a similar nearby neighborhood continued its pattern of high emergency room utilization.[63]

The health center programs have been the greatest effort to date in the battle against inaccessibility to primary care. They have been remarkably effective in reaching target populations. An average of 66 percent of eligible individuals and 55 percent of all eligible families in the target areas used services at the health centers. Some centers reached as many as 93 percent of the eligible families and 97 percent of eligible individuals in the target area.[64] Unfortunately, their effects have been difficult to evaluate with precision because every access problem was tackled simultaneously, and "before and after" measures at the same sites using the same variables were not collected. Therefore, a definite answer about the relative importance of each access factor will not be forthcoming.

Factors Influencing Access to Primary Care

Although increased attention has been focused on barriers to access during the last ten years, particularly for those living in poverty, certain ones continue to limit the use of primary care.

1. *Barriers relating to site and its location.* Consumers tend to use services within an idiosyncratic "circle," the outer perimeter of which is determined by distance, time, and energy. *Within* that circle, how one person selects among available services is not related primarily to distance, but to other factors such as the manner in which one is treated by providers, the language spoken, one's feeling of acceptance and familiarity, and other elements influencing personal preference. At times, however, these factors influencing selection may be such that usage is effectively blocked or the patient is forced to go beyond his "radius of convenience." For example, psychological barriers can interfere, as in the case of a group of aged women in Oakland, California who reported that the two greatest barriers that kept them from medical care were fear of being mugged and fear of stray dogs. In another example, West Oakland residents, probably because of sociocultural or informational barriers, failed to consider obtaining care at nearby "Pill Hill," a concentrated block of hospitals and private physician offices standing on the edge of the ghetto and where many were eligible to receive services under the Medicaid program. Instead, they complained about the great distance they had to travel to the county hospital clinic.[65]

Beyond the circle, utilization is more likely to decrease directly as distance, time, and energy expenditures increase. Most studies show that as distance increases, the services used, especially preventive services, tend to decrease.[66] To go far afield to illustrate this point, Bryant reports a study from Uganda showing that when patients have to travel over one hour to reach services, utilization decreases by one-half.[67] Patients in this country are no different. For many groups in the United States, the time getting to services is inordinately long.[68] Bellin and Geiger[69] reported that 14 percent of Columbia Point residents spent five hours or longer, and an additional 70 percent spent from two up to five hours, door-to-door to obtain medical care prior to the development of the OEO health center. In Watts, the phrase "$10 sick" referred to the fact that to get to the county hospital across town took hours on the bus. To avoid such a trip required ten dollars for the taxi. Only when one was "really sick" was this trip made.[70]

Usage may be altered simply by the conditions of roads (winter versus summer), or by having to spend time and energy to circumvent a freeway, a railroad, or a canyon standing between the patient and primary care. The patient's own condition may create energy expenditures he can ill afford. If a man is old and incapacitated or if a mother has to carry two children and lead three others, the patient may not be able to go any distance at all.

Patient perceptions about the appropriateness of these time/energy expenditures are also relevant. One hour on foot or in a jeep over almost impassable roads, or one hour on a crowded bus may serve as a marked deterrent for those who are not sure whether preventive pediatric care serves any purpose. The suburban mother, on the other hand, may accept the necessity of spending 40 to 50 minutes on the freeway and 10 to 15 minutes finding a parking space near the pediatrician's office because her concept of distance and time has been altered by her expectations and experience, and by her acceptance that well-baby care is an essential service.

In an attempt to overcome barriers related to site location, most health centers under OEO have been placed as centrally as possible in the catchment area served. In Watts, for example, 43 percent of the regular users could walk to the center[71]; in Rochester, 69 percent.[72] Elective and preventive services may need to be even closer to the patient than those used for acute illness. For this reason, health departments have traditionally placed well-baby clinics in the neighborhood. Following this example, health center systems, like the one in Denver, have created neighborhood outpost stations[73]; and clinical nursing centers for continuing supervision of persons with chronic diseases have been set up in Memphis close to the homes of the chronically ill.[74] Decentralization has been particularly necessary in rural primary care programs. The Beaufort-Jasper program, for example, has five small subcenters scattered throughout the two counties, making care more accessible to all.[75]

In any situation, there will be those who do not live within walking distance and are without transportation. This percentage will be higher in programs caring for large numbers of poor. In Watts, 6 percent need transportation to health services[76]; in Rochester, 11 percent.[77] When ruralness is added to poverty, more usage of special transportation facilities can be expected. In the King City Rural Health Program in California, approximately 30 percent use the little "red bus"[78]; and in Beaufort-Jasper, despite decentralization of facilities, over 80 percent are reported to need transportation.[79]

The ultimate in making the site of services convenient to the patient is through house calls and telephone contact. As providers have become busier, more harassed, and more efficiency minded, care in the home has become less and less common in the United States. House calls now constitute a small minority of patient contacts. For example, a study in upstate New York[80] found that only 4 percent of the visits of general practitioners were to the home. This figure was 5.6 percent in a study conducted in Massachusetts.[81] By contrast, in England, 20 percent of patient visits are still provided at home, and physicians spend considerable parts of their day in "domiciliary" care.[82] This curtailment in the United States has apparently been accepted as a *fait accompli* by consumers, even though they often complain bitterly about it.

Little effort has been made by providers to analyze whether house calls still serve an important function for certain persons and families. Information about the physical and social environment of the patient's home can only be collected by such a visit. House calls also play an important role in the development of trust between providers and patients. Patients visited in their homes relate afterwards in a much more personal way to providers, accepting their advice and help with less hesitancy. Similarly, providers seem to develop greater rapport with and understanding for the patient. However, the most important role of house calls remains that of placing the service conveniently for the patient—particularly for those who are aged or chronically incapacitated and who find it difficult, if not impossible, to negotiate the distance to the office or clinic, even when transportation is available.

Increasing access through the telephone is another important way to overcome distance. Although it has been widely used by the private sector for entry, triage, and treatment, it has received little attention by other types of primary care delivery systems. Yet, if creatively used, it can greatly diminish barriers in the way of service. In the Los Angeles County-University of Southern California Medical Center diabetic program,[83] nurse practitioners known to the patients were made available by telephone around the clock. In this way, patients could easily obtain advice, get their prescriptions filled, and make appointments for future visits. Not only was the convenience of the patient served, but a consequent reduction in hospitalization saved the county large sums of money.

2. Barriers because of the time services are available. Service hours are an important factor in underutilization, and noticeably so in creating "distorted" utilization patterns by some groups, e.g., the use of emergency rooms for nonemergent conditions. Hours when care is available are decided by providers, not patients. However, the most acceptable time for patient use of services may be quite different from the time most convenient to providers.

It is interesting to note the peak utilization hours that emerge when service times are broadened. Health centers under OEO, usually open between 9 a.m. and 9 p.m. and on Saturday mornings, experienced two peak utilization periods—one in the morning and one in the early evening. This fact suggests that there are two utilizing groups with dissimilar needs, and that traditional times for care—whether in clinics or private offices—may not serve the "after-hours" utilizers.

Individuals in any care system, no matter how flexible its hours, will still get sick in the middle of the night and on Sunday when the regular staff is off duty. Most of us are familiar with the bind that occurs when we begin to realize how sick a family member is after 10 p.m. First, there is the reluctance to bother the provider; then the wait until worry supersedes reluctance; the difficulties in negotiating beyond switchboard operators or telephone answering services; and finally, if no physician can be reached, the trip to the emergency room. This process is difficult and trying for the affluent with a personal physician. For the poor, it may be impossible.

To solve such problems, utilization peaks must be determined for any group served. If indicated, the hours of services need to be enlarged or shifted, and for the occasional late night and weekend calls, a skeleton staff with access to records and back-up providers must be easily reachable, at least by telephone.

3. *Financial.* Most attention by health policy makers has been directed to financial factors. This is appropriate, for inability to finance health care has in the past, and still today, limited or excluded many families from obtaining primary care services. Primary care is the place, after all, where care is most likely to be delayed, where it can be eliminated if there is a financial squeeze, where insurance benefits are least likely to apply, and where other measures—such as home remedies—may be substituted.

While Medicaid and Medicare programs have in recent years markedly decreased the discrepancies in per capita physician visits per year among different socioeconomic levels, the gap has not been closed completely. Financial factors cannot be forgotten, particularly when one considers access to primary care. Many of the poor do not qualify for Medicaid or live in states where benefits are minimal. Those covered by Medicare still experience differences in the use of services on the basis of income.[84] The adverse effect of coinsurance and deductibles, especially devastating for low-income groups and one of the operative factors in creating discrepant Medicare benefits, was clearly demonstrated in Scitovsky's and Snyder's study where the introduction of a 25 percent coinsurance provision in a comprehensive prepaid plan for medical care substantially reduced the demand for physician services.[85] Finally, those with no insurance, in particular those who live just above the poverty level with little disposable income, are often caught in the tightest bind of all.

Up to now, I have discussed access in terms of what the primary care organization can do. In the case of financial factors, however, an organization has little ability to effect change. Only a national program of health insurance covering low-income families with copayments kept at a minimum, or the direct provision of accessible and acceptable services with no cost to the patient can broaden financial accessibility for the medically indigent.

4. *Organizational factors.* Although system factors are repeatedly cited as creating difficulties in access, there is little documentation of their impact. Long waiting times, difficulties in making appointments, impersonal treatment, little regard or sensitivity to cultural characteristics, frequent change in physicians and nurses, complex bureaucratically oriented policies, demeaning eligibility procedures, a maze of buildings and clinics to be navigated, fragmented services, no clearly identifiable entry procedures, and the inability to reach a provider when needed are some of these organizational factors. Too few primary care systems, whether they be clinics or private offices, have been aware of the effect their behavior has on utilization. Individual and institutional providers alike have had the attitude of sellers with the market tied up: "Take it or leave it; that's the way it is."

Organizational change need not involve large expenditures of money or time. Much can be done by a change in provider attitudes and a sensitization to the needs of the patient. I am not implying that change can be easily accomplished. Physicians seem to have a particularly hard time in changing professionally learned behavior. Yet, it is possible to alter systems so that people are treated with dignity and respect. It is possible to handle health care information confidentially. It is possible to provide translators, perhaps on a voluntary basis when funds are not available. It is possible to clearly identify services, to tell people about them, to explain how to get in the system, and to open the doors literally and figuratively. To make change in these ways, however, takes professional leadership and vision and involvement of consumers to point out how conditions, no longer apparent to professionals, limit care.

Those in lower socioeconomic brackets, those who come from minority backgrounds, the aged, and those living in remote and isolated regions face the greatest limits to primary health care. These are the very groups who have the least influence on how care is delivered. This observation provides some indication as to why access factors of all kinds have received little consideration by health providers in the past. When consumers were allowed to take part in program planning and development, as in the OEO health center programs, they placed major emphasis on facilitating care, and actively sought to eliminate organizational characteristics that mitigated against its use.

5. *Patient factors.* Social and cultural factors, as well as personal characteristics associated with age, sex, and past experience, play important roles in determining how patients will use primary care—both through the realities of life that such conditions impose and by the way they influence consumer knowledge, attitudes, and practice. Many research studies have demonstrated this relationship between patient factors and utilization behavior.[86]

Patients may not recognize the existence of health problems. They may not believe that their own condition warrants health care services. They may have no sense of urgency or may place little value on receiving care (particularly if physicians use unintelligible language or provide what seems to be irrelevant information). I have met many consumers who feared to go for medical services because they believed that they would be the subject of experimentation. I have spoken with others who found the health care organization alien and hostile or believed that it had connections with police or immigration authorities inimical to their own future safety. I have seen pride keep a mother from taking her children to the clinic until they could all be perfectly dressed with clean clothes, and I have seen husbands who would not allow their wives the liberty of attending a clinic alone.

In considering how patient factors limit access, primary care organizations have too seldom responded by seeing the need to change their own behavior. More often they have attempted to see if they could change the patient. Perhaps less attention should be paid to patient values and attitudes as a guide for *patient* change, and more attention paid to them as a guide for *organizational* change.

The "hard to reach" have something to tell provider systems and we should listen.

I would suggest three responsibilities that primary care systems should assume in order to reduce access problems. First, with the participation of consumers, clean their own houses so that system factors creating negative attitudes in patients are ameliorated and that organizational characteristics are compatible with the social and cultural expectations of patients. Second, make certain that patients have *full information* about health, available health services, and how they can be used. In particular, information must be provided about entry, how patients can best use the system, and why and how confidentiality is handled. Third, whenever possible, tackle problems that directly prevent the use of services by patients,[87] e.g., organize babysitting pools, acquire translators, provide transportation, be open at convenient hours, or recruit volunteers to sit with the aged.

Issues around the Comprehensiveness of Services

Earlier in this section I discussed the way in which primary care tasks are carried out by different types of primary care organizations, the quantity and distribution of primary care providers, and the barriers to existing services. Throughout this discussion certain issues around the comprehensiveness of services have surfaced. The creation of new primary care arrangements and systems will require policy makers and health planners to grapple with substantive aspects of these issues, such as 1) how broad the scope of services will be, 2) whether new health-oriented and community approaches missing from primary care today will be incorporated, and 3) whether essential services now provided by separate subsystems and by public health agencies will be integrated into primary care systems. I would like to address these issues in somewhat greater detail.

What Should the Breadth of Services at the Primary Level Be?

The first question to be asked is, "To what extent are primary care systems responsible for ensuring a comprehensive breadth of services for their patients?" I have previously discussed seven categories into which possible services can fall: 1) outreach; 2) entry, triage, and referral; 3) clinical/technical interventions (and auxiliary services); 4) human support; 5) patient education; 6) facilitation; and 7) coordination. It must be made clear that these are the services needed by *groups*; an individual or a family unit will never need all of them—even over a lifetime. Groups on the other hand, if composed of a substantial number of members that represent a cross section of society by socioeconomic level, sex, and age, will require the full range of services over a period of time. Comprehensiveness, therefore, is a *system* attribute and it is in this context that we must view it.

Health professionals, when viewing such a list of comprehensive health care services, usually say, "This would be utopia. No system could possibly include them all." I believe that this reaction is a product of the way we have been trained to think. We are not accustomed to thinking that we have a responsibility to groups, nor that all the elements entering into the process of care are an integral part of the whole. To avoid this bias inherent in the "health professional culture" dominated by physicians, it is necessary for each service system to go beyond the traditional criteria of comprehensiveness. In so doing, it may be necessary to involve consumers in analyzing the process of care as it is they who can best tell us what services are required in order for patients to understand the need for care, gain access to it, and utilize it.

Although services offered will obviously vary according to the particular health, patient, and environmental needs of a population, all primary care systems need to expand beyond their present narrow medical focus. I would like to discuss in a little more detail some of these areas of expansion. The *outreach function,* for example, has not usually been part of health care services. For the most part, patients have initiated health care when they have recognized a health need (present or future), or when they have desired other types of benefits (e.g., human support) that can be obtained only by declaring themselves sick. This is a perfectly appropriate way for most patients to use the system. For others, however, particularly those living in poverty, the health system may need to reach out in a more active way. Yet, once the patient is introduced to care, a continuing outreach function *per se* may or may not be required.

As health systems develop prepaid contracts, patients will need to be enrolled, either as individuals or groups. Here, the concepts of "marketing" for enrollment and "outreach" overlap. "Marketing" may have acceptance in an ever-increasing, efficiency-minded industry whereas the broader "outreach" will not. This, in my opinion, would be a great misfortune as the outreach component can play an important role in providing information, building trust, and acting as the adjudicator of discrepant professional-consumer viewpoints.

Even in the case of the *clinical/technical services,* gaps currently exist between the model and the actual practice of primary care. This is due to the fact that certain services are not considered necessary by many medically oriented providers, and because these providers do not believe that the health problems of an individual must be treated in the context of the family and community. But knowledge of issues pertaining to a patient's health needs is required beyond that obtained in the usual medical history, and new ways must be developed to obtain it, to develop family record systems, and to create new contacts with the community.

Also, when an individual's health problem is the result of an environmental situation inimical to his health, which is particularly common among poverty groups, primary care must be concerned with the elimination of the cause as well as alleviating its effect. For example, if water is contaminated, patients must be advised about alternative actions they can take. Services might include instructions about how to dig, encase, and seal a new well, and in some programs the manpower to dig the well might even be provided. This type of "comprehensiveness" is a far cry from seeing a physician for 10 to 15 minutes in an ambulatory facility.

Support services for persons around times of birth, death, mental breakdown, and incapacitating illness are fast diminishing with the change and disappearance of institutions that once provided them. As the extended family vanishes and the numbers of children decrease, fewer family members are available to be of assistance to each other. The church has become inaccessible to many. Self-contained communities with helping neighbors are being swallowed up and deformed. Many people have few places to turn for support when emergencies overwhelm them or when crises of lesser magnitude still loom large in their lives. Social casework services are insufficient for this function and are not readily accessible nor acceptable; mental health systems are often rejected because people are reluctant to be categorized as "mentally sick."

Primary care has traditionally been expected to provide these support services, but as private practitioners have become busier and practice settings have altered, they seem less able to see "support" as a legitimate responsibility and less able to respond to patient needs in this respect. The need of patients for human support combined with the increasing inability of primary care providers to provide it is one of the major reasons, I believe, for the current disparity between patient and provider expectations. The importance of "high quality" medical care based on scientific and technological excellence is generally accepted by patients. In addition, what they often want, however (but do not state), is someone who cares, who relieves anxiety, who provides some support through the pain and turmoil of life, and who gives advice and help as well as "scientific ministrations." This constant frustration may underly much of the consumer discontent expressed in complaints of "too long waiting," "too impersonal," "no house calls," and "can't find a doctor." Although these complaints are valid and based on reality, they may also be manifestations of resentment of providers who do not listen nor support.

Educational services are another area which health professionals have recognized as important but have done little to integrate into the ongoing continuum of primary care. Five methods of health education are possible: 1) a provider, on a one-to-one basis, may work with a patient (or family member) around issues directly affecting his or her health; 2) a patient may be provided with information in written or audio-visual form; 3) classroom instruction, such as prenatal classes, can be arranged; 4) group process may be used to forward behavioral change; or 5) large groups of patients may be reached by mass media techniques. Health programs have focused attention on the latter four in settings such as hospitals, health departments, and voluntary health agencies. Unfortunately, they have not been available, to any large degree, as part of primary care.

The one-to-one educational process between a primary provider and a patient has received even less attention. All providers are supposed to "educate," and many, especially physicians, believe that they are uniquely qualified for this task. In the actual primary care setting, however, little regard has been paid to how information is transmitted, how the patient may best be able to internalize it, and whether time is allowed for its inclusion (e.g., short patient visits allow little time for education). In contrast, child health conferences using public health nurses have typically employed a more structured approach to education. Perhaps as we move toward the use of nurse practitioners and pediatric associates in primary care, educational services will be improved. Also, where consumers have a continuing relationship with groups of providers—as in health centers, in prepaid group practices, and in the general practitioner groupings evolving in the United Kingdom—more intensive and extensive patient education programs become a feasible endeavor.

It is in the realm of *coordinative services,* in my opinion, that primary care as presently organized fails most severely by too seldom providing for effective coordination and continuing management of patient care. Two types of coordination are needed: the first links services over time; the second links and monitors all personal health care services taking place in the present, whether auxiliary to primary care or at the secondary or tertiary levels. At present, many patients must serve as their own coordinators and patient care managers, and they must do this without training, ongoing supervision, or an assisting record system. Continuity and management require a system in which an easily accessible and retrievable record accompanies the patient and allows for contributions from multiple providers, and they also require the assignment of the patient to a specific provider group which assumes ongoing responsibility for his care.[88]

Should Primary Care Systems Include More Health-Oriented Activities?

Health and disease are socially and culturally determined concepts, and in our western society have been viewed as a single continuum with health at one end and overt disease at the other—health being the absence of, or opposite of disease. The personal health care system, in line with this concept, has focused on disease and its prevention. Even health promotive and preventive activities are, for the most part, focused on potential pathological states—e.g., immunizations, seat belts, or education about smoking.

There is another way to look at health and disease, however, that allows them to be separate although interlocking phenomena. The World Health Organization defines health somewhat in this way as "a state of complete mental, physical, and social well-being and not just the absence of disease and infirmity."[89] Audy,[90] taking this concept further, views health and disease as existing on entirely separate continua. From this viewpoint, health can be defined as an individual's ability to rally from insults or as the process of maintaining homeostatic balance with the environment, and health is, therefore, theoretically a separate entity and potentially measurable. In other times and in other cultures, health has been defined in this way. Hellenistic and Oriental cultures have had elaborate philosophical or religious systems which have sought to describe the interdependence of mind, body, and environment and to discover techniques for maintaining the balance between them. It is interesting to note that today's "counter-culture" also places significance on becoming healthy through attention to diet, exercise, massage, and state of mind.

Curiously, but perhaps predictably, as people become healthier, they also become more interested in health-focused activities. In the United States today many of the more affluent classes seem addicted to the search for health. They patronize the health food store; they jog; they take vitamins in large doses; they develop new institutions, such as the "health maintenance organization" in Berkeley which for a yearly prepayment will provide families with "health services" rather than medical care.[91]

In spite of this growing consumer interest in the idea of health as a separate entity, it has not been incorporated to any great extent into primary health care.[92] There are several reasons for this. First, we have few tools by which to measure health and little systematic or scientific knowledge about its production. Second, we do not train providers to deal with their patients' concerns about "healthy" living. Providers tend to see themselves as scientists interested only in the empirically verifiable and the "curable." Finally, throughout history man has focused first on the immediate—what is hurting, what makes him sick, what kills him. He has not been allowed the luxury, except in rare circumstances, to think about what he might become. The United States, however, may be approaching a stage of development in which more people can afford to be concerned with being healthy.

Some primary care services, going primarily to mothers and children, are the exception and relate directly to health rather than to disease. For instance, prenatal programs which provide the prospective mother with information about proper diet and exercise during pregnancy and offer training in exercises to facilitate labor and delivery are specifically health-oriented, as are many infant care activities such as nutritional advice and developmental guidance.

Although most action influencing health must continue to come from outside of the health system itself—from changes in the way people live, in the food they eat, in their housing, their income level, their transportation, their exercise, their stress, and their daily patterns of life—I believe primary care could do more than it is doing and should expand its activities around health maintenance as distinguished from disease prevention. Implicitly, primary care is being asked to do just that by increasingly large segments of the population who are turning to health food stores and faddists.

Should Primary Care Systems Take Part in Organized Activities to Change Community Situations Causing Health Problems?

A primary care system that cares for an identifiable population, whether defined by enrollment or geography, is in an unusual position to contribute directly to health status improvement by organized activities other than the delivery of personal health care services. It is uniquely able to understand the conditions affecting its clients' health, and because of its valued services, it is easier for a primary care system to gain the trust and esteem of the community than it is for health departments or other community agencies. This trust makes it easier to work with community groups, a required ingredient for community change.

Neighborhood health centers have pioneered in attempting to stretch the meaning of primary care in this direction. They have fostered community action and education programs around better housing, food supplements, legal attacks on obstacles to health, increased social services for patients, waste disposal systems, and community drug control.

Primary systems developed in the future should accept the challenge of this more broadly defined concept of health care and consider whether or not they wish to become so involved.

Should Other Subsystems of Personal Health Care Be Integrated into or Coordinated with Primary Care Systems?

As I previously discussed, providers from a variety of disciplines have developed separately functioning subsystems with few linkages to each other. Recently, however, as the idea of integrated primary care has experienced increased acceptance, prepaid plans and neighborhood health centers have often included dental, optometric, and mental health services as part of their benefits. Those negotiating prepaid Title XIX contracts in California, for example, are now grappling with strategies for the inclusion of the services of several subsystems into their benefit packages.

Even in optimally integrated settings, traditional patterns of "apartness" prevail. The first director of OEO's Comprehensive Health Services Division, a dentist by background, wanted to see the fullest possible integration of dental services into health center programs. Common patient care records were to be used; the dentist and the paradental staff were to be part of the primary care team; and the inclusion of dental chairs in each team area was urged. A few health centers attempted to integrate to this extent. Most, however, clung to the norms of the outside world and designed independent dental units. Even so, this was a great step forward. Services were in the same facility. Prescriptions from both physician and dentist could be filled at a common pharmacy. Common records gave dental workers access to information about the patient's home and history. The same family health worker could assist with entry, and dentists could turn to the family health worker to follow up missed appointments. The same transportation system could be used, and the same telephone number and the same complaint mechanism were available.

There is little doubt that primary care would be greatly enhanced if the integration of its various subsystems could be accomplished. It remains to be seen whether old separatist patterns can be overcome to create an efficient, high-quality, cohesive whole.

Should Services Now Provided under the Auspices of Health Departments Be Integrated into Primary Care Systems?

Primary care systems, moving toward "comprehensiveness" and toward "health maintenance," may hesitate to include certain outreach, coordinative, facilitiative, and human support services in their programs because of the increase of immediate costs and the lack of evidence, as yet, of their ultimate financial impact. I would suggest that some of these services are already available and primarily being paid for by public funds and that the consumer, because of organizational fragmentation, is not getting his money's worth.

In 1968, more than 20,000 public health nurses were employed by the over 2000 local health departments and 600 visiting nurse services.[93] Although public health nurses also assume responsibility for community activities such as disease control and school health programs, the tasks of primary care make up much of their daily work. They serve as unsung health care coordinators, helping to maintain continuity of care for many of the poor who receive highly fragmented and less than adequate primary care services from public clinics, emergency rooms, or private practitioners. In addition, public health nurses help families get to care, educate, follow up physician instructions, and assist in the solution of family and environmental problems.

It is a great waste of money and energy for the two parts of the primary health care team[94] —the physician in the office and the public health nurse in the field—to make so little attempt to work closely together. As it is now, they do not share patient *groups* in common, they possess no common records, and they only rarely communicate on a regular basis with each other. In most situations the public health nurse, while intimately involved with family care, is not recognized as a viable or legitimate team member, either by the physician or dentist. Sometimes they do not even know of her existence.

With the development of new primary care systems, the opportunity exists to create a marriage between these independently functioning providers. An important demonstration in this regard is taking place in Great Britain where primary care has been traditionally assigned to the general practitioner. There, many general practices are undergoing evolutionary changes leading them toward a new primary care model. Small group practices are increasing in number and many are moving into health center configurations. By 1971, 1292 general practitioners (6.5 percent of all general practitioners in England and Wales) were expected to practice out of 225 health centers.[95]

More important for our discussion, however, a move has been made to consolidate the components of the primary health care team—the general practitioner, the public health nurses (health visitors), and the nurses responsible for bedside nursing care (district nurses). The latter two are being assigned by the local health department (medical officer of the local health authority) to work full time out of the general practitioners' offices or centers.[96] "Health visitors," for example, may handle such primary care services as house calls, follow-up visits, and bedside care. They may provide promotive and preventive services such as well-baby clinics, prenatal care classes, and group educational sessions in the general practitioner's office. In some cases, they are performing clinical duties at the middle level of practice.[97] In a few situations, local social workers have also been deployed to the general practitioner's office to deal with health problems that clearly must be treated in the context of the patient's social environment. The general practitioner's office has been described as a good "pick up" point for social casework with the social worker being able to serve as a personal link between the physician and district social services.[98] In Britain, therefore, a primary health care team, offering a broad range of services in a nonfragmented manner supported by public finances, is slowly emerging and moving toward reality.

It is now feasible for us to begin to think along similar lines with the assignment of public health and visiting nurses, full or part time, to organized primary care programs. Because it is the nature of organizations to part reluctantly with their responsibilities, this process may go slowly. Public health agencies are no more flexible than other organizations in this regard, as I learned when developing health centers for OEO where attempts to persuade health officers to assign public health nurses to health centers often met with resistance. Nevertheless, it is essential that organized primary care programs, such as those involving medical foundations or small physicians' groups with prepaid Title XIX contracts, integrate the *services* of such workers into their delivery mechanism.

DIRECTIONS FOR THE FUTURE

There are overriding human and financial reasons why the long neglect of the primary level of health care should end.[99] In charting a course for change, however, it is no longer sufficient to react to problems alone. These are only the visible symptoms created by deep-seated deficiencies. It is to the basic structure of the primary care system that attention must be directed.

I have shown diagrammatically in Figure 9 how problems and deficiencies of primary care are manifestations of structural arrangements embedded in a social and cultural environment that emphasizes individualism, both in patient behavior and system response. It is not my intent that this exercise would be exhaustive or complete; rather it is an impressionistic attempt to illustrate a *process* that helps to identify underlying structural deficiencies. Because all of these involve multiple and intricately interlocking relationships, simple solutions will not suffice.

Some of the structural arrangements, most of which I have touched on previously in this paper, are:

- Responsibility for the personal health care of population groups is unassigned and therefore unassumed.
- No regulatory apparatus exists to define and ensure basic primary services for patient groups.
- Organizational   structures   necessary   for   planning,   continuity,

FIGURE 9
LINKAGES BETWEEN PREDISPOSING SOCIAL AND CULTURAL ENVIRONMENTAL FACTORS, STRUCTURAL ARRANGEMENTS, AND PRIMARY CARE DELIVERY PROBLEMS

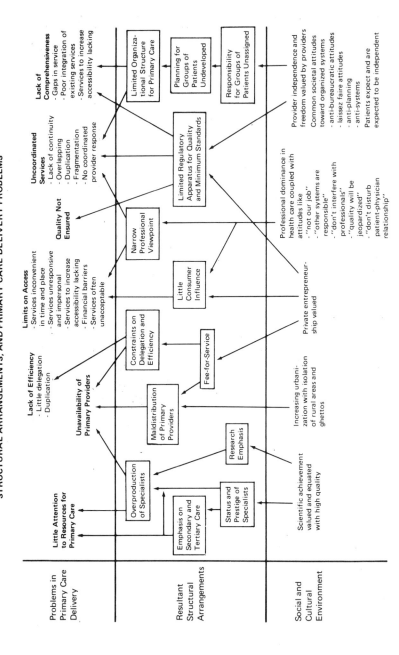

coordination, and comprehensiveness of primary care do not exist.

- Financial reimbursement systems make increased efficiency of care, introduction of new workers, and other necessary changes difficult to achieve.
- Professional dominance, with little input from consumers, has shifted health services in the direction of science and technology and away from personalized care.
- Professional dominance, with little input from consumers, has resulted in little attention to accessibility issues.
- Emphasis by educational institutions on the quality of scientific and technical achievement as opposed to the delivery of care has produced providers with little interest or ability to function in primary care situations.[100]

Assignment, regulation, new organizational arrangements, reimbursement mechanisms that do not constrain innovation, increased consumer involvement—these are the directions in which change must proceed.

The change will no doubt be evolutionary and pluralistic in nature, and the diversity of the models already beginning to appear suggests that the massive development of a system built around a single model, whether we call it a health maintenance organization or a neighborhood health center, is unlikely. I also believe a single model is undesirable. Patients and providers both need the opportunity to link themselves with systems that best fit their particular needs. In addition, those desirable aspects of present health care delivery, particularly the personalized relationships possible in private primary practice, must not be totally lost but must have the opportunity to be incorporated into more adequate and responsive organizations.

We can probably expect widely varying systems to develop, ranging from loose confederations of office-based primary practitioners operating under the aegis of county medical foundations to highly centralized Kaiser-like systems; from programs with professional sponsorship to ones that are consumer controlled; from small units enrolling ten to twelve thousand persons and providing only basic primary care services to those serving millions and including all health subsystems and all levels of care; from centralized urban programs to far-reaching rural systems. Yet, however varied the arrangements may be, I hope there will be a general conviction that the ultimate product needs to be similar—coordinated and comprehensive services delivered by providers sensitive to the needs of patient groups and accountable to them.

We must appreciate that the reorganization of primary care cannot be viewed only from the "here and now." Solutions launched today or tomorrow may not be fully realized for five, ten, or even fifteen years. It is now eight years since the first neighborhood health centers were funded under OEO, and we have not begun to clarify the lessons learned; ten years or more may be needed to understand that endeavor and others like it. Since we have to plan so far ahead, we must anticipate as much as possible, the attitudes and demands of those who will be the consumers of services in the next twenty years.

Throughout, I have espoused the importance of making consumer needs and wants the highest priority when planning for and making decisions related to health care. This is essential if systems are for consumers rather than providers. I suspect that from now on we will be forced to think more in these terms for I believe that the patients of the future will be more aware, more sophisticated, and more determined to have a health system that meets their needs. They will continue in the age-old search for the "healer," but they will expect this "healer" to combine scientific and technical know-how with "caring." Their knowledge about health and disease will continue to grow and with it a demand for more involvement in the process of care and the "demystification of medicine." As overall health status continues to improve, they will become less disease-oriented for much of their life span, expecting to have more "health" measures provided. And increasing longevity and numbers of older people will create a demand for long-term, continuous patient-provider relationships.

The complexity of making the needs of future patients compatible with those of future providers, and out of that amalgam producing effective and efficiently delivered primary care services, is almost overwhelming. But the fact that changes in primary care will have an impact far beyond the primary level of care lends urgency to our task of restructuring. To use an architectural analogy, primary care is the *keystone* of the arch of personal health care. Without it in place, the structure of the health care system has no stability; the other components of the arch cannot effectively serve their particular functions, and the *personal* health care system as a total entity will remain distorted, costing too much, delivering too little, satisfying too few.

REFERENCES

1. Mechanic, D., Some Notes on the Future of General Medical Practice in the United States, *Inquiry*, 6, 17-26, June, 1969.

2. See the following references for other definitions of primary care:

    American Medical Association, Council on Medical Education, Ad Hoc Committee on Education for Family Practice, MEETING THE CHALLENGE OF FAMILY PRACTICE, Chicago, September, 1966.

    The Citizens Commission on Graduate Medical Education (John S. Millis, Chairman), THE GRADUATE EDUCATION OF PHYSICIANS, Chicago, American Medical Association, 1966.

White, K. L., Primary Medical Care for Families—Organization and Evaluation, *New England Journal of Medicine,* 277, 847-852, October 19, 1967.

Division of Health Care Services, Community Health Service, A CONCEPTUAL MODEL OF ORGANIZED PRIMARY CARE AND COMPREHENSIVE COMMUNITY HEALTH SERVICES, Rockville, Maryland, U.S. Public Health Service, U.S. Department of Health, Education and Welfare, 1970.

British Medical Association, REPORT OF THE WORKING PARTY ON PRIMARY MEDICAL CARE, Planning Unit Report No. 4, London, B.M.A. House, May, 1970.

The Role of the Primary Physician, A Report on the Conference on the Role of the Primary Physician in Health Services, *WHO Chronicle,* 25, 567-573, December, 1971.

Brunetto, E. and Birk, P., The Primary Care Nurse—The Generalist in a Structured Health Care Team, *American Journal of Public Health,* 62, 785-794, June, 1972.

Fry, J., Information for Patient Care in Office-Based Practice, *Medical Care,* 11, 35-40, Supplement, March-April, 1973.

3. One must distinguish between ambulatory and primary care for they are not synonymous. Many ambulatory patients are receiving secondary level services (e.g., cobalt therapy), and many bedridden patients in nursing homes and extended care facilities remain under primary care management.

4. Parker, A. W., THE TEAM APPROACH TO PRIMARY HEALTH CARE, Neighborhood Health Center Seminar Program Monograph Series Number 3, Berkeley, California, University Extension, 1972.

5. These have been described as nonintensive, low-specialization, and majority services by DHEW in A CONCEPTUAL MODEL OF ORGANIZED PRIMARY CARE AND COMPREHENSIVE COMMUNITY HEALTH SERVICES, *op. cit.*

6. This follows the problem-oriented approach of Larry Weed which, it seems to me, is as applicable when used with this broader definition of clinical/technical interventions as it is when limited to medical care alone. (MEDICAL RECORDS, MEDICAL EDUCATION, AND PATIENT CARE: THE PROBLEM-ORIENTED RECORD AS A BASIC TOOL, Cleveland, The Press of Case Western Reserve University, 1969.)

7. Here I should like to make a distinction between the pharmacist as a *direct instrument* of primary care—i.e., when he performs a triage and referral function or institutes care such as providing an ointment for a poison oak dermatitis; and when he serves as an *auxiliary*—i.e., fills a prescription and instructs the patient in its use.

8. Jeffreys, M., AN ANATOMY OF SOCIAL WELFARE SERVICES, London, Michael Joseph, 1965.

   Fry, J., PROFILES OF DISEASE, London, E. & S. Livingstone, Ltd., 1966.

9. Fink, D., *et al.,* The Management Specialist in Effective Pediatric Ambulatory Care, *American Journal of Public Health,* 59, 527-533, March, 1969.

10. Parker, A. W., *op. cit.*

11. Suchman, E. A., Social Patterns of Illness and Medical Care, *Journal of Health and Human Behavior,* 6, 2-16, Spring, 1965.

12. National Center for Health Statistics, PHYSICIAN VISITS—VOLUME AND INTERVAL SINCE LAST VISIT, UNITED STATES, 1969, Vital and Health Statistics, Series 10, Number 75, Washington, D.C., U.S. Department of Health, Education and Welfare, July, 1972.

13. Recent statistics indicate that there are approximately 2500 outpatient departments and 5500 emergency rooms,[a] 30 prepaid group practices,[b] 150 comprehensive health centers,[c] and 200 free clinics.[d]

    (a) National Center for Health Statistics, HEALTH RESOURCES STATISTICS, HEALTH MANPOWER AND HEALTH FACILITIES, 1971, Rockville, Maryland, Department of Health, Education and Welfare, 1972.

    (b) Richardson, E. L., Statement before the Health Maintenance Organizations Hearings, Subcommittee on Public Health and Environment of the Committee on Interstate and Foreign Commerce, House of Representatives, 92nd Congress, April 11, 1972.

    (c) U.S. Office of Management and Budget, THE BUDGET FOR FISCAL YEAR 1973, SPECIAL ANALYSES OF THE U.S. GOVERNMENT, Washington, D.C., Government Printing Office, 1972. (Figure represents the 1973 estimate of OEO comprehensive health care projects and HEW partnership for health centers.)

(d) American Medical Association, Council on Medical Service, Committee on Health Care of the Poor and Committee on Community Health Care, Statement on Free Clinics: 1972, Chicago, November, 1972.

14. For a general discussion and evaluation of neighborhood health centers, see Langston, J. H., *et al.,* STUDY TO EVALUATE THE OEO NEIGHBORHOOD HEALTH CENTER PROGRAM AT SELECTED CENTERS, Rockville, Maryland, Geomet, Inc., January, 1972.

For a specific example of the attempt to implement a holistic approach, see the Dr. Martin Luther King, Jr. Health Center, FIFTH ANNUAL REPORT, Bronx, New York, 1971.

For a review of quality in health centers, see Morehead, M. A., Donaldson, M. S. and Seravelli, M. R., Comparisons between OEO Neighborhood Health Centers and Other Health Care Providers of Ratings of the Quality of Health Care, *American Journal of Public Health,* 61, 1294-1306, July, 1971.

15. Collen, M. F., Research with a Defined Population, in THE KAISER-PERMANENTE MEDICAL CARE PROGRAM, Proceedings of a Symposium, Oakland, March, 1971, A. R. Somers, ed., New York, The Commonwealth Fund, 1971, pp. 129-137.

16. For example, Kaiser in Portland and Fontana (Calif.), Group Health of Puget Sound (Renton Center), the Harvard Community Health Plan, and a private group practice in King City (Calif.) have had grants enabling them to enroll disadvantaged groups and to use family health workers.

17. Hurtado, A. V., *et al.,* The Utilization and Cost of Home Care and Extended Care Facility Services in a Comprehensive, Prepaid Group Practice Program, *Medical Care,* 10, 8-16, January-February, 1972.

18. Riley, G. J., Wille, C. R. and Haggerty, R. J., A Study of Family Medicine in Upstate New York, *Journal of the American Medical Association,* 208, 2307-2314, June 23, 1969.

19. OEO has recognized these potential resources and has provided developmental grant monies to a number of outpatient clinics, such as County-University Hospital in San Diego, San Francisco General Hospital, Boston City Hospital, and the New Jersey College of Medicine and Dentistry.

20. American Medical Association, Statement on Free Clinics, *op. cit.*

21. Torrens, P. R. and Yedvab, D. G., Variations among Emergency Room Populations: A Comparison of Four Hospitals in New York City, *Medical Care*, 8, 60-75, January-February, 1970.

California Medical Association, Bureau of Research and Planning, SURVEY OF EMERGENCY AND DISASTER MEDICAL SERVICES, San Francisco, December, 1969.

Jacobs, A., *et al.*, Emergency Department Utilization in an Urban Community, *Journal of the American Medical Association,* 216, 307-312, April 12, 1971.

22. Lavenhar, M. A., Ratner, R. S. and Weinerman, E. R., Social Class and Medical Care: Indices of Nonurgency in Use of Hospital Emergency Services, *Medical Care,* 6, 368-380, September-October, 1968.

23. If there were no primary physicians in the United States, we could say that primary physicians were unavailable. But if there should be one in San Francisco and one in New York, primary physicians could be considered available, but inaccessible because of the distances involved, and the fact that each would have to care for 100 million people. This exaggerated picture is given only to point out how difficult it is to separate these two concepts as I am using them.

24. American Medical Association, DISTRIBUTION OF PHYSICIANS IN THE UNITED STATES, 1971, Chicago, 1972. For this discussion I am only using the count of office-based physicians even though hospital-based physicians contribute a considerable percent to the total of primary physician visits. The reason for this exclusion is the difficulty in developing full-time equivalents for primary care for interns, residents, and full-time staff members, all of whom devote part of their day to secondary level care or training activities.

25. Fry, J., MEDICINE IN THREE SOCIETIES, New York, American Elsevier Publishing Co., 1970.

26. It is difficult to arrive at exact measures of the percent time that pediatricians and internists spend in primary level care. Schonfeld has used percent of patients referred to them in order to derive this figure (NAPS Document 01733, New York, National Auxiliary Publications Services, 1972). Using Schonfeld's method, the percent of time spent at the primary level can be estimated at 76 percent for internists and 95 percent for pediatricians in 1968 (based on figures from the National Disease and Therapeutic Index, Specialty Profile, Ambler, Pa., Lea Associates, Inc., 1972). Clearly, percent referred is not identical with secondary and tertiary level care, but I think it approximates actuality.

27. In 1931, physicians were classified as being in private practice. In 1971, the classification included all physicians practicing in an office.

28. The 1931 average utilization of physician services was 2.5 per capita, and by 1969 it had risen to 4.3. (The Committee on the Costs of Medical Care, FINAL REPORT: MEDICAL CARE FOR THE AMERICAN PEOPLE, Chicago, University of Chicago Press, 1932; and National Center for Health Statistics, PHYSICIAN VISITS, *op. cit.*)

29. Those in general practice in the U.S. in 1970 saw an average of 172.9 patients per week, while those in internal medicine saw 122.6 and pediatrics, 145.2. The number of hours per week spent in direct patient care averaged 47.7, 45.5, and 45.9 respectively. (American Medical Association, REFERENCE DATA ON THE PROFILE OF MEDICAL PRACTICE, Chicago, 1972.)

30. American Medical Association, DISTRIBUTION OF PHYSICIANS IN THE UNITED STATES, 1969, Chicago, 1970.

31. National Center for Health Statistics, PHYSICIAN VISITS, *op. cit.*

32. American Medical Association, SELECTED CHARACTERISTICS OF THE PHYSICIAN POPULATION, 1963 and 1967, Chicago, 1968.

33. Robertson, L. S., On the Intraurban Ecology of Primary Care Physicians, *Social Science and Medicine,* 4, 227-238, August, 1970.

34. Because of the difficulties in arriving at acceptable ratios, and the problems inherent when ratios are compared between different parts of the country and between rural and urban areas, their use was abandoned and it was decided instead to use locally derived designations of "scarcity" based on such indicators as the quantitative lack of resources, inaccessibility, and ineffective utilization.

35. Crystal, R. A., Health Manpower Scarcity Areas and Their Characteristics, Presentation made before the Task Force on the Manpower Distribution Project of the National Health Council, Memphis, January 24, 1973.

36. Ferguson, L. A., What Has Been Accomplished in Chicago?, in MEDICINE IN THE GHETTO, J. C. Norman, ed., New York, Appleton-Century-Crofts, 1969, pp. 87-97.

37. Haynes, M. A. and McGarvey, M. R., Physicians, Hospitals and Patients in the Inner City, in MEDICINE IN THE GHETTO, J. C. Norman, ed., New York, Appleton-Century-Crofts, 1969, pp. 117-174.

38. American Medical Association, Counties without an Active Physician in Patient Care, in DISTRIBUTION OF PHYSICIANS IN THE UNITED STATES, 1971, *op. cit.,* pp. 12-16.

Fahs, I. J. and Peterson, O. L., Towns without Physicians and Towns with Only One—A Study of Four States in the Upper Midwest, 1965, *American Journal of Public Health,* 58, 1200-1211, July, 1968.

39. Jefferson County-Pine Bluff Health Center, Comprehensive Health Services Application, Pine Bluff, Ark., May 1, 1970.

40. Fendall, N. R. E., Primary Medical Care in Developing Countries, *International Journal of Health Services,* 2, 297-315, May, 1972.

41. Schonfeld, H. K., Heston, J. F. and Falk, I. S., Numbers of Physicians Required for Primary Medical Care, *New England Journal of Medicine,* 286, 571-576, March 16, 1972.

42. Lee, R. I. and Jones, L. W., THE FUNDAMENTALS OF GOOD MEDICAL CARE, Chicago, University of Chicago Press, 1933.

43. The difference between Schonfeld's count of 120,000 and the 1971 figure of 84,099 in Table II is due to the fact that he included hospital-based physicians in primary specialties, unspecified specialties, doctors of osteopathy, and a percentage of the work performed by obstetricians and gynecologists, while I have simply counted office-based general practitioners, general pediatricians, and general internists.

44. Members supplementing care outside the plan must also be considered in looking at physician-population ratios in prepaid group practice plans.

45. It is interesting in this regard to look at the United Kingdom where the average number of persons carried by one primary physician on his panel can be determined. By 1968, the ratio was 1:2477 for the country as a whole, with some 44 areas where physicians were having to care for panels of over 3200. (British Medical Association, REPORT OF THE WORKING PARTY ON PRIMARY MEDICAL CARE, *op. cit.*)

46. Golden, A., Associate Professor and Director of the Health Associate Program, School of Health Services, Johns Hopkins University, Baltimore, Personal Communication, June 8, 1973.

47. Dorsey, J., Harvard Community Health Plan, Personal Communication, June, 1973.

48. Mason, H. R., Manpower Needs by Specialty, *Journal of the American Medical Association,* 219, 1621-1626, March 20, 1972.

49. Fahs, I. J. and Peterson, O. L., The Decline of General Practice, *Public Health Reports,* 83, 267-270, April, 1968.

50. Recently, an almost explosive development of family practice residencies has occurred. The new specialty was officially recognized in 1969. By the end of that year, 22 residencies had been approved, increasing to 62 in 1970, 103 in 1971, and 170 at the present time. The chairman of the American Board of Family Practice, Dr. Nicholas J. Pisacano, believes optimistically that within a decade, 30 to 40 percent of all physicians graduated will go into family practice. He projects a continued increase in residencies and the production of several thousand family practitioners annually by 1980. (Personal Communication, June 4, 1973.)

51. National Academy of Sciences, NEW MEMBERS OF THE PHYSICIAN'S HEALTH TEAM: PHYSICIAN'S ASSISTANTS, Report of the Ad Hoc Panel on New Members of the Physician's Health Team of the Board of Medicine, Washington, D.C., 1970.

52. The extensive use of mid-level providers to take over tasks now assigned to physicians raises the question of where these physicians, after long years of training, will fit into primary health care in the future. Three configurations seem possible. 1) They could continue to carry the responsibility for most primary care tasks, delegating only a few to the physician assistant or nurse practitioner, e.g., well-baby supervision, triage, or management of patients with chronic disease. This seems to be the common pattern emerging. 2) The physician assistant or nurse practitioner could be given a much larger share of primary care tasks, the physician being retained to provide supervision, consultation, and final decision making (perhaps only in the strictly medical area of health care), therefore extending his services to much larger populations. 3) The physician could move toward the management role as described by John Bryant (HEALTH AND THE DEVELOPING WORLD, Ithaca, Cornell University Press, 1969), in which he serves as "team leader," acting not only as a supervisor, consultant, and medical decision maker, but also responsible for the total health and well-being of a specific population or enrolled group. This role for primary physicians, although not uncommon in developing countries, is not yet a valid one in this country except to a limited extent in the health center movement.

53. Mason, H. R., Effectiveness of Student Aid Programs Tied to a Service Commitment, *Journal of Medical Education,* 46, 575-583, July, 1971.

Fenderson, D.A., Major Problems of Health Manpower Maldistribution, Presentation made before the Task Force on the Manpower Distribution Project of the National Health Council, Memphis, January 24, 1973.

54. Bible, B. L., Physicians' Views of Medical Practice in Nonmetropolitan Communities, *Public Health Reports,* 85, 11-17, January, 1970.

55. Steinwald, C., Factors Influencing the Distribution and Location of Physicians: Literature Review, in American Medical Association, DISTRIBUTION OF PHYSICIANS IN THE UNITED STATES, 1971, *op. cit.,* pp. 25-31.

56. A National Health Service Corps staff member informed me that eleven out of twenty-three of those placed in one region have signaled their intent to remain. (Galiher, C., Personal Communication, May 17, 1973.)

57. Cook, W. H., Profile of the Permanente Physician, in THE KAISER-PERMANENTE MEDICAL CARE PROGRAM, *op. cit.,* pp. 97-105.

Tilson, H. H., Characteristics of Physicians in OEO Neighborhood Health Centers, *Inquiry,* 10, 27-38, June, 1973.

58. The question of personal satisfaction is a very crucial and complex one. Physicians are trained for autonomous action, and as presently socialized, a sense of responsibility and sense of control are essential to them. Unless or until physicians can be trained for satisfaction through interdependency and shared responsibility, the practice environments must take the need for autonomy into consideration.

59. Stanford Research Institute, CHIROPRACTIC IN CALIFORNIA, Los Angeles, The Haynes Foundation, 1960.

60. Medical Committee for Human Rights and the California Council for Health Plan Alternatives, Feelings about the Kaiser Foundation Health Plan on the Part of Northern California Carpenters and Their Families, Report to the Carpenter Funds, San Francisco, April 5, 1973.

61. South Central Multipurpose Health Services Corporation, Health Center Services Survey, A Study of Patient Perceptions of Selected Service Areas and Other Aspects of Patient Care and Patient Utilization, Los Angeles, undated.

62. Roghmann, K. J., Haggerty, R. J. and Lorenz, R., Anticipated and Actual Effects of Medicaid on the Medical-Care Pattern of Children, *New England Journal of Medicine*, 285, 1053-1057, November 4, 1971.

63. Hochheiser, L. I., Woodward, K. and Charney, E., Effect of the Neighborhood Health Center on the Use of Pediatric Emergency Departments in Rochester, New York, *New England Journal of Medicine*, 285, 148-152, July 15, 1971.

64. Langston, J. H., *et al., op. cit.*

65. West Oakland Health Center, Application for 314(e) Health Services Development Grant, Appendix C, Survey undertaken by West Oakland Health Council, Inc., 1967.

66. Weiss, J. E., Greenlick, M. R. and Jones, J. F., Determinants of Medical Care Utilization: The Impact of Spatial Factors, *Inquiry*, 8, 50-57, December, 1971.

67. Bryant, J., *op. cit.*

68. The time-cost to the individual includes *two* travel times (back and forth), waiting time, visit time, and prescription-filling time. According to the 1969 National Health Survey, the average length of time for a patient to get to the doctor's office was 17.2 minutes. When added with the other times, the average visit cost is 1½ hours of patient time, while a visit to a hospital outpatient clinic averages two hours.

69. Bellin, S. S. and Geiger, H. J., The Impact of a Neighborhood Health Center on Patients' Behavior and Attitudes Relating to Health Care, *Medical Care*, 10, 224-239, May-June, 1972.

70. English, J. T., Office of Economic Opportunity Health Programs, *Inquiry*, 5, 43-48, March, 1968.

71. Leyhe, D. L., Gartside, F. E. and Procter, D., MEDI-CAL PATIENT SATISFACTION UNDER AN OEO NEIGHBORHOOD HEALTH CENTER AND OTHER HEALTH CARE RESOURCES IN SOUTH CENTRAL LOS ANGELES, Medi-Cal Project Report No. 4, Los Angeles, University of California School of Public Health, March, 1972.

72. Hillman, B. and Charney, E., A Neighborhood Health Center: What the Patients Know and Think of Its Operation, *Medical Care*, 10, 336-344, July-August, 1972.

73. Cowen, D. L. and Sbarbaro, J. A., Family-Centered Health Care—A Viable Reality?, *Medical Care*, 10, 164-172, March-April, 1972.

74. Runyan, J. W., Jr., *et al.*, A Program for the Care of Patients with Chronic Diseases, *Journal of the American Medical Association*, 211, 476-479, January 19, 1970.

75. Barnwell, T., Project Director, Beaufort-Jasper Comprehensive Health Services, Inc., Personal Communication, August 9, 1973.

76. Leyhe, D. L., Gartside, F. E. and Procter, D., *op. cit.*

77. Hillman, B. and Charney, E., *op. cit.*

78. Huerta, V., Administrator, Rural Health Project, King City, Calif., Personal Communication, June 5, 1973.

79. Barnwell, T., *op. cit.*

80. Riley, G. J., Wille, C. R. and Haggerty, R. J., *op. cit.*

81. Brown, J. W., *et al.*, A Study of General Practice in Massachusetts, *Journal of the American Medical Association*, 216, 301-306, April 12, 1971.

82. Riley, G. J., Wille, C. R., and Haggerty, R. J., *op. cit.*

83. Miller, L. V. and Goldstein, J., More Efficient Care of Diabetic Patients in a County-Hospital Setting, *New England Journal of Medicine*, 286, 1388-1391, June 29, 1972.

84. Davis, K., Financing Medical Care: Implications for Access to Primary Care, Paper presented at the Sun Valley Forum on National Health, Sun Valley, Idaho, June 28, 1973.

85. Scitovsky, A. and Snyder, N., Effect of Coinsurance on Use of Physician Services, *Social Security Bulletin*, 35, 3-28, June, 1972.

86. Aday, L. A., THE UTILIZATION OF HEALTH SERVICES: INDICES AND CORRELATES, A RESEARCH BIBLIOGRAPHY, Lafayette, Indiana, Health Services Research and Training Program, Department of Sociology, Purdue University, R. L. Eichhorn, Director, 1972.

McKinlay, J. B., Some Approaches and Problems in the Study of the Use of Services—An Overview, *Journal of Health and Social Behavior*, 13, 115-152, June, 1972.

87. It must be remembered that the groups with the most acute access problems tend to constitute a minority of those served. If health care systems wish to consider these issues, they must, therefore, decide how much time, effort, and money should be spent to develop special services for small groups. These decisions will be especially critical in the prepaid setting, where the cost could conceivably be spread to all members. While the principle of shared risk is accepted for medical conditions, it is foreign to issues of access.

88. Professionals in health care speak of "continuous" versus "episodic" use of services. However, from the patient's perspective, his own health care is always continuous; it always relates to what went on in the past and what will occur in the future. It is important that the health system he is part of sees him in the same way as he sees himself and that it is capable of maintaining a continuous, coordinated response to his needs. The patient can then turn to it *as* he sees fit, perhaps only occasionally, which the provider may see as "episodic." This is the patient's prerogative.

89. WHO, First Ten Years of the World Health Organization, in ANNEX I, CONSTITUTION, Geneva, 1958.

90. Audy, J. R., Measurement and Diagnosis of Health, in ENVIRON-MENTAL: ESSAYS ON THE PLANET AS A HOME, P. Shepard and D. McKinley, eds., New York, Houghton Mifflin, 1971, pp. 140-162.

91. The Center for the Study of Health Maintenance Practices, Your Neighborhood Health Maintenance Center, Berkeley, California (2018 Blake St.), undated brochure.

92. Interestingly, services provided by the neighborhood health centers, with few exceptions (e.g., infant care, prenatal care, family planning), have been disease-oriented. This is understandable. Health centers serve populations beset with disease and disability. Treatment and prevention of disease are the highest priorities. The search for health in positive terms is a luxury available only to those who are healthy and have the time to make an effort to pursue it—a middle class phenomenon in our society. Free clinics for this reason have been less inhibited, often stressing the importance of health and the necessity of being responsible for one's body. Even there, however, it seems health professionals and their disease-oriented thinking have tended to dominate the scene.

93. American Nursing Association, FACTS ABOUT NURSING, A STATISTICAL SUMMARY, 1970-71 Edition, New York.

94. The assignment in some health departments of certain traditional public health nursing tasks to new workers from the community is beginning to create a "community-oriented" team, consisting of a public health nurse with family health workers, which is able to reach patients in ways unavailable to professional office-based workers.

95. Curwen, M. and Brookes, B., Health Centres: Facts and Figures, *The Lancet,* 2, 945-947, November 1, 1969.

96. Anderson, J. A. D., *et al.,* Attachment of Community Nurses to General Practices: A Follow-up Study, *British Medical Journal,* 4, 103-105, October 10, 1970.

    Dixon, P. N. and Trounson, E., Evaluation of Health Centre Community Nurse Team, *British Medical Journal,* 1, 306-309, February 1, 1969.

97. Smith, J. W., Extended Use of Nursing Services in General Practice, *British Medical Journal,* 4, 672-674, December 16, 1967.

98. Goldberg, E. M., *et al.,* Social Work in General Practice, *The Lancet,* 2, 552-555, September 7, 1968.

99. The experience of prepaid plans and certain medical foundations leaves little doubt that utilization at the secondary and tertiary levels of care can be decreased by more appropriately controlled services at the primary level. In the meantime consumers are caught in a "Catch-22." The more they spend at the secondary level, either as individuals or collectively as a nation, the less they have available to spend on primary care. At the same time, the less they spend on primary care, the more they are forced to spend at the secondary level. This cycle needs to be broken.

100. Primary care also has another grave deficiency. It has no one group that is able to serve as its advocate for promoting the development and maintenance of primary care systems. This is in contrast with both the secondary level (with hospital and specialty groups) and the tertiary level (with strong research and academic ties).

ACKNOWLEDGMENTS

The preparation of this paper has been partially supported by OEO grant #90037(b). I wish to thank all the members of the Health Center Seminar Program staff for their invaluable assistance, especially Jane Walsh and Sumiyo Kastelic for their editorial help. I am particularly grateful to Catherine Petersen for providing much of the documentation.

DISCUSSION

ROBERT J. BLENDON: Three points, I think, might place Alberta Parker's paper into perspective.

First, we need to recognize that the problem of an inappropriate national mix of physician specialists (too many surgeons, too few primary care physicians) is not synonymous with the problem of poor geographic distribution of physicians in general. Unfortunately, the evidence suggests that solving the first problem will not likely resolve the second.

The United States is faced with a unique public policy problem in the health area. It comes about as a result of an economic phenomenon rarely seen in a market-oriented society such as ours. That is, physicians are able to create their own demand for services. This phenomenon permits them to select the places where they will practice regardless of the actual need for their services. By varying their fees or volume of services rendered per patient, physicians can choose practice locations without having to suffer the economic consequences of such decisions.

This relates to the American system of health care financing. It means that regardless of the number of physicians the country produces, little can be expected in physician settlement patterns. Because physicians are now able to concentrate their practices in favored geographic localities, any efforts to change the mix of physician specialists and generalists alone will have little impact on the geographic distributional system. The net effect of shifting medical graduates away from medical and surgical subspecialties into primary care training programs would be to leave us with a situation in which the suburban housewives of the country would be over-doctored by family practitioners instead of surgical and medical subspecialists as is currently the case.

How physicians can so influence their geographic location is seen in a comparison of New York State with a ratio of 228 physicians per 100,000 people to Mississippi with 82 physicians per 100,000. This occurs in spite of the fact that the rate of new medical students graduating is increasing faster in the state of New York than in the state of Mississippi. The same problem can be seen in Massachusetts. With eight million people Massachusetts can, without any economic hardship, support the same number of neurosurgeons as Great Britain which has 55 million people.

In my view, there is no evidence that primary care practitioners (general practitioners, general internists, general pediatricians, and family practitioners) will settle differently than other specialists. In fact, a study in Baltimore tracing trends of physician settlement over a decade showed that primary care practitioners were more likely to leave the inner city than their specialty colleagues.

Given then this unique phenomenon, that physicians can and do control demand for their services, the specialty choice of a physician becomes only one factor in affecting his settlement decision. The other factors, I believe, are economic, cultural, technological and, for lack of a better term, law and order.

Second, we need to recognize that rural and inner city physician scarcity problems are fundamentally different issues. This is particularly important when we consider educational training programs as one possible avenue for remedying the problem.

In terms of resources, rural and inner city communities often look the same because the current system measuring physician office locations often misses the hidden system of secondary physician care which exists in the inner cities of most metropolitan areas. What is not measured by current statistical practices are the numbers of physicians in training or full-time physicians on the staffs of medical schools or publicly owned hospitals. These institutions, in fact, provide the bulk of the care available to most inner city populations. This error in counting the availability of services in cities gives the erroneous impression that in inner city census tracts, there are no ambulatory care services available. This is not the case. By simply looking at the poverty area surrounding the Johns Hopkins Hospital east of Baltimore the miscount becomes obvious. The Johns Hopkins Hospital; although unlisted as a center for private practice, provides almost 500,000 ambulatory care visits annually. In terms of serving the city of Baltimore alone, this figure would equal one out of seven physician visits provided within the city.

This capacity of providing ambulatory care services is missed in the statistical counts because it is provided by a team of almost 500 physicians in training, plus a hundred part-time and full-time backup medical faculty members whose office locations are either in the suburbs or in the medical school. The important point here is not that a hidden system of providing secondary care (cardiology, ENT, psychiatry, general surgery and specialty pediatrics) actually exists at these hospitals, but rather that any physician practicing in the inner city independently of such an institution must only have the skill levels required to render frontline, primary care services.

By contrast, in rural communities the statistical count is quite accurate and available health services not only suffer from a lack of primary care providers but also of secondary care specialists. In rural areas, because of the low geographical density and the need to maintain 24-hour-a-day coverage seven days a week, primary care physicians not only need skills for frontline care duties, but they also must be prepared to provide some basic secondary care and to handle most nonsurgical emergencies.

The use of physician extenders has been suggested in this regard. But it can only be partially successful in this rural environment because of the need for coverage for secondary care which prohibits use of physicians' assistants in the absence of backup of a secondary care physician.

The problem of having to have primary care provided in rural areas by practitioners who also have secondary skill levels is, I believe, one of the most compelling rationales for family practice training programs in this country. Because of the randomness of secondary care needs in rural populations, training individuals who cannot cope with basic secondary care problems along with the provision of primary care will in no way provide a system capable of maintaining the minimal needs of rural America.

In discussing the scarcity of physicians in rural areas, it is popular these days to place the blame on medical schools. According to this misconception, many rural communities do not have physicians because medical schools stopped training general practitioners. This is not quite true. The disappearance of office-based medical practice occurred because of far more important economic and cultural reasons. We often fail to realize that the development of the city with its metropolitan area corresponded to the same time period that scientific changes were occurring in medicine. It led to the general belief that since medical schools were concentrating on the training of physician specialists, many rural communities lost their opportunity to have physicians. In my opinion the loss of physicians in rural America occurred independently of physician specialization. The play of other factors was so strong that regardless of the trends occurring in medical education, this country still would have faced a physician maldistribution problem.

My third point relates to a political issue. The fact that physicians can and do create their own demand for services is an extraordinarily difficult problem to resolve within the American political process.

As I see it, the United States is a country with a heavy psychological dependence on the free market concept as an instrument for resolving most distributional problems. There is substantial evidence that in the field of medicine the market is not functioning particularly well. However, we are so addicted to the concept, that I see a future of government attempts to keep spinning the same dials by trying to improve the situation through manipulation of the market place. Given the nature of the system and the control physicians exercise over it, such efforts by the government are likely to be quite expensive and lead to very few distributional changes.

Recognizing the problem does not in any way mean that we as a nation will be unable to deal with it adequately. . . . The national response, however, will not likely be the same in regard to the training of physician specialists. Almost half of the funds for medical education are now provided by the federal government. Likewise, there has been a history in the science field of federal planning for scientific manpower. The precedent of public sector involvement in higher education will provide a precedent for more active intervention. To borrow a phrase from Governor Wallace, "We're going to send them a message." Given the chronic problem of an inappropriate mix of physician specialists, I see by the end of the decade the federal sector utilizing its financial leverage on medical schools. The only remaining issue will be, not whether the message be sent, but rather, what will it say when the medical schools receive it?

CHAPTER 2 • CHARLES E. LEWIS

Improving Access to Primary Care Through Reforms in Health Education, Orientations, and Practice

Once upon a time, just before one of the great wars to end all wars (1940 to be exact), the United States had a health care delivery system primarily populated by providers of primary care. There were 133 practicing physicians per 100,000 population and 62 percent of them were in general or primary practice. A significant proportion of physicians were located in communities of less than 50,000 population. Less than 10 percent of the people in the United States at that time were covered by any form of health insurance, and the average rate of hospitalization was 74 per 1,000 individuals per year. The average life expectancy at birth was 62.9 years.

Three decades later, let us examine what progress has been made. The current physician-population ratio is 153 per 100,000 and only 19 percent of physicians in practice are classified as family or general or primary care practitioners. Eight and two-tenths percent of physicians practice in communities of less than 50,000. An increased proportion of the population, almost 90 percent, is covered by some form of health insurance, the number of hospitalizations has almost doubled (145/1,000 persons/year), and the expected length of life of a child born in 1970 was 70.8 years.

Since the title of this chapter contains the word "reforms" and one of the definitions given for reform is "to restore to former goodness," it might be implied that a nostalgic approach to the solution of the problem of access to primary medical care would be to turn back the clock by reconstructing the kinds of institutions—schools, hospitals, etc.—with which we achieved former "goodness," as reflected in the statistics cited. Obviously, this argument falls into the category of *reductio ad absurdum* and we are left with suggesting alternate solutions.

I assume that one way in which a complex and differentiated health care "system" can increase its functional effectiveness is the development of appropriate organizational schemes and *management* mechanisms that assure communication and integration among the various specialized fragments. A second approach is somewhat related to the "return to former goodness" for it requires a core of generalists competent in assessing the problems of individuals on first contact with the "system." The generalists who represent the interstitial glue and perform the major distributive function in this type of organization require two sets of abilities: first, the ability to deal with a majority of the problems presented, independently of the rest of the organization, and secondly, to be able to identify and refer those who need further service. To perform this latter function the generalists must have *access* to specialists, technical resources, facilities, etc. It is not always fully appreciated that consumers are not the only ones who have problems with "access" within the health care system. One of the forces related to the reduction in the number of generalists is *their* problem in gaining "access" to the rest of the system.

Doctor Bergen's chapter elsewhere in this book has dealt with solutions that involve the first alternative; that is, more effective organization and management of a complex system. A discussion of the means of generating and distributing the generalists or primary care providers constitutes the first part of this paper. Other alternatives involving educational processes such as teaching consumers how to "beat the system" or how to avoid it, constitute the concluding section.

For someone who has been intimately involved in the process of medical education for almost 25 years (the first 1/3 as subject, and the remainder as observer-experimenter) an opportunity to discuss the variables that influence the output of medical education provides both an occasion to summarize a great deal of highly fragmented and generally non-generalizable data, as well as to ventilate my frustrations as both subject and researcher—although I shall try to minimize this aspect of the presentation.

While there is a great deal of "information" in the literature on medical education, very little knowledge has been systematically collected about the workings of medical education.

DISTRIBUTION BY CONTENT OF PRACTICE

I should like to propose the following over-simplified model for the analysis of the output of medical education: A dependent variable, "Y_s," indicates the specialty or type of practice selected by the medical graduate. The independent variables include the following:

1. The characteristics of the student admitted to medical school:
    (a) basic intelligence,
    (b) performance in certain undergraduate courses,
    (c) sociocultural background, including the social class of his (or her) family, ethnic group, and size of their home community.
2. The structure of the curriculum, including the types and quantity of specific subjects taught, and the sequence in which various content

areas are presented to the student. (We might also add the extent to which *real* electives are provided, and the nature of the true grading system–pass/fail, letter grade, or numerical rating.)

3. The nature of the role models provided by faculty members who transmit both information and values to the novitiate.

4. The value systems held by both the students and faculty members (here I have specific reference to what kinds of subjects are important/unimportant, what kinds of behaviors are valued/not valued, what are the dimensions of excellence?).

5. Societal values or inducements. These include differential earnings by type of specialty, as well as society's image of "different" kinds of physicians–Marcus Welby versus Ben Casey.

6. The student's spouse, i.e., the majority of students now come to medical school with an additional asset and determinant of future plans. The social class of their wife's/husband's family, the size of her/his home community, expectations/needs and personality are part of this equation.

7. The options open to the student as a graduate, in terms of kinds of internships and residencies available, where they are located, in what specialties, how much they pay, etc., as well as further graduate opportunities such as traineeships, fellowships, etc., must be considered.

8. Finally, to this list of independent variables one must add an error term and pray that it is randomly distributed.

Before commenting on what we know about each of these variables from existing data, it is only fair to point out that since no studies have been conducted that have considered all of these, we have no estimates of the r^2, or total amount of variance in the dependent variable that might be accounted for by all of these factors.

It has been demonstrated that the best predictor of "success" in a medical school (as measured by graduation) is the student's undergraduate grade point average in the "hard sciences."[1] Since most of the attrition in medical education occurs during the first two years, and since the basic science courses are based upon and are taught in the model of the undergraduate "hard science courses" this might be considered as constituting one of the many self-fulfilling prophecies that permeate this field.

A variety of studies have demonstrated that personality or noncognitive characteristics are associated significantly with the selection of certain types of medical specialties. Demographic factors,[2,3] cognitive styles of decision-making,[3] personality characteristics,[4,5] and social values[5] have been demonstrated to be associated significantly with selection of type of practice. In the past more general practitioners have come from lower class family backgrounds, from smaller communities, and could be stereotyped as more pragmatic, action-oriented, more "rigid" and less concerned with abstract concepts or contemplative problem-solving activities. At the other end of these multidimensional spectra are those selecting careers in psychiatry and public health. It is impossible to summarize this literature in a few sentences, but despite the differences in methodologies and design certain commonalities emerge. One study has even demonstrated certain "risk factors" associated with "social activism" in medical students.[6]

The citations listed in this chapter do not represent an exhaustive review of the literature on personality characteristics and career selection. Schofield has recently published an annotated bibliography of "Research Studies of Medical Students and Physicians Utilizing Standard Personality Instruments" containing 51 references.[7]

Even the order of exposure to certain content areas can affect attitudes. In our favorite laboratory (the University of Kansas), it was demonstrated that sequences of third-year clerkships (assigned randomly to students) were associated significantly with the acquisition of patient-centered versus disease-centered orientations.[8] It was also possible to demonstrate that certain kinds of curricular "innovations" such as introducing students to a multi-disciplinary team approach to care of chronically ill patients in their homes during the first year of medical school, reinforced the learning of the basic sciences related to clinical medicine, as well as created a "patient-centered" orientation.[9] (However, given exposure to the rest of the curriculum, all evidences of this particular "treatment" had disappeared within two years.) We also documented the futility of introducing certain kinds of cross-disciplinary teaching models as late as the fourth year of medical school.[10]

There has been considerable discussion, but very little experimentation, regarding the importance of "role models." In the absence of hard data we can only assume that the importance of modeling behavior, as demonstrated in other areas of education, holds for medicine also. Some of the concerns expressed by those promoting the creation of departments or divisions of family practice are that medical students are educated by specialists and never exposed to family practitioners as members of the faculty, and that most of the diseases studied by medical students are not reflective of the content of primary care.

With respect to importance of values held by peers and faculty, there are also little data available. One piece of evidence that might be offered is a study by us (unreported) of the geographic distribution of graduates of the University of Kansas Medical School according to rank in class. Rank in class may be considered to be some sort of function based upon the aptitude of the student, plus faculty judgments based on their views of "excellence" in medicine. For graduates of the University of Kansas during the years 1930 to 1950 there was an inverse relationship between rank in class and the probability of practicing within the state. In other words, the majority of those who graduated near the top of their class did not end up practicing in the state. One can only speculate that current practices prevailed whereby the "best" are recruited by internships and residencies at "elite" university hospitals. In contrast, the majority of those who graduated in the lower ranks of their class took rotating internships and went into primary care, frequently in small communities within the state that had supported most of the costs of their medical education.

Data on the values of society as they affect the dependent variable in this model are also scarce. One study has examined choice of specialty on the basis of economic returns to the physicians.[11] A more interesting variable (at least to some of us engaged in this type of research) is the impact of the wife of the medical student on access to care. Data from a study of medical student-couples at the University of Kansas suggested that over 50 percent of all medical students believed that their wives were significant determinants of their choice of a type of medical career. In the same study, over 90 percent of the wives indicated the same beliefs.[12] Wives based their reasons for "directing" their husbands into specific types of practices (notably away from primary care, general or family practice) on the basis of having talked to Dr. X's wife: "It's obvious that while he makes a lot of money, he has no time to spend with his family. What's the good of having all that money if you don't have any time to spend it?" As will be indicated later, there is even stronger evidence that wives are significant determinants of the size of community in which their physician-husbands decide to practice.

While the continued reference to studies of the *wives* of medical students/physicians may be interpreted as evidence of the male chauvinism rampant in medical education, the absence of any discussion of the impact of "female" medical students/physicians represents a statistical reality rather than a covert error of omission. Studies of the impact of spouses on decision-making cited were conducted at a time when women represented less than 6 percent of all medical students and active practicing physicians in the United States; also at that time the overwhelming majority of young women physicians/medical students were unmarried.

The increasing representation of women among entering classes in medical schools in the United States may have a positive impact on the availability of primary care physicians. The United States has fewer women physicians than any other developed/overdeveloped/developing country in the world, and many have suggested that the mixture of curing/caring/coping functions required of the primary physician might well be performed more effectively by women. (These remarks are not intended to suggest that women physicians are not sufficiently competent to become internists, neurosurgeons, etc.)

The options for postgraduate training available depend on the "market," on the student, and his recommendations from the faculty (their estimates of his "excellence") as well as the kinds of institutions looking for specific kinds of medical graduates. As indicated by Miller, students select medical schools just as medical schools select students.[13] This same joint decision-making process applies to postgraduate education. Students who graduate with "honors" may do so because they are "junior" versions of the faculty. Perhaps research findings from elementary education apply to medical education as well. These findings suggest that children who are physically attractive do better academically,[14] and there is a significant association between "academic performance" as judged by the teacher, and the extent to which the student is "supposed" to do well as determined by prior testing.[15] I suspect (without proof) that this is quite true in medicine. The extension of this possibility to its ultimate conclusion is that the "best" doctors become involved in research/teaching and specialty medicine and that the others (by inference, the less competent) can't get into the prestigious institutions for postgraduate training. Therefore, they end up either taking specialty training in "lesser" institutions or else settle for a career in "primary practice." I believe this value judgment may represent the most significant variable in the equation.

GEOGRAPHIC DISTRIBUTION

Since it is impossible to discuss access in terms of number of specialists and generalists without considering their geographic distribution, it seems appropriate to generate a similar model that might be used to describe the spatial distribution of physicians.

In this equation, the dependent variable ($Y_{location}$) is related to the following: (1) some measure of the economic wealth of an area such as per capita income or personal disposable income; (2) the supply of physicians already present in the area; (3) the location of the site of postgraduate training of the physician; (4) the nature of the home community of the physician; (5) the nature and size of the home community of the physician's wife; (6) personal values (desire for a certain climate, recreational facilities, etc.); (7) technical requirements related to certain types of practices, i.e., the need for certain hospital resources; and (8) organizational requirements, i.e., the fact that some medical specialties require a rather large patient population because of the infrequency of "conditions" seen by that specialty.

Reviews of the literature examining many of these factors have been conducted by several individuals including Fein, Butter, etc.[16-19] They might be summarized as indicating that the economic resources of an area along with the site of postgraduate training seem to be the best predictors of physician distribution. There is little evidence that physicians tend to go back to "where they came from"; therefore, the recruitment of physicians from inner-city or rural areas is not a very potent predictor of a propensity to return to serve in that area.* Perhaps of equal importance to the physician's origins are those of his spouse. In a study of over 1,000 practicing physicians in Kansas in 1968, the generalization could be made that physicians did not practice in communities smaller than those in which their wives grew up. In other words, almost every physician practicing in a community of less than 10,000 was married to a woman who spent her early childhood in a community that size.[20]

---

*A recent report from Illinois takes exception to this statement.

Before examining the implication of these models in terms of solutions of access to primary care, it should be noted that almost all activities in medical education are based on the principle that *the individual has free choice to do what he wants to, where he wants to, regardless of who has paid for his education.* To repeat, the principles of a democratic society are seen as applying to both the specialty and geographic distribution of medical manpower.

Let us consider what could be changed within the immediate future, i.e., within a few years, in the equation describing the distribution of physicians. Those of us who have had considerable experience in the organizational activities of medical schools (faculty curriculum committees, executive committee activities, etc.) would suggest that neither the curriculum nor the role models will be changed very rapidly (thanks to tenure). If the faculty do not change, then the values held by the faculty (and their organization) also will be relatively immutable. It is also improbable that societal values will change rapidly, and unless the institution of marriage disappears completely, any attempt to provide premedical students exposure to a specific set of women might be considered beyond the limits of human experimentation. The only variables reasonably susceptible to change relate to the characteristics of those admitted, and subsequently the values of the peer culture of medical schools. But what happens if we mix new kinds of students with old kinds of faculty? There are very few experiments of this type and none have occurred intentionally, to my knowledge. However, we might conclude from some of the observations made in the late 1960s during the advent of "radicalism" in medical school or from more recent policies to admit students with different kinds of undergraduate backgrounds or from different social groups that, in general, students are expected to adapt to the organization and the expectations of the faculty, rather than the reverse, . . . or else.

In all probability the characteristics of students admitted, given "reasonable" evidence of intellectual ability, could influence the output of medical schools. It is also probable that *major* reforms in curriculum could have a significant impact. Medical education is based on what could be described as the inverted pyramid curriculum, which begins with the provision of basic science information and terminates with the student selecting a specific type of career, and then *relearning* the basic sciences relevant to that specific specialty. If students were provided some minimal basic science content and then required to select a specific career in pediatrics, primary care, surgery, etc., a more logical restructuring of the rest of the curriculum could occur. In almost all medical schools there is *no* statement of the *objectives* of the medical school in terms of what kinds of practitioners they will graduate, except generalities such as "physicians capable of problem solving, and willing to pursue a lifetime of learning, intelligent, adapting, brave, clean, . . . "

Many programs developing intermediate health workers such as nurse practitioners and physicians' assistants are based upon the second approach. Some have begun by writing specific educational objectives, i.e., defining the scope of practice of their graduates, and have constructed curricula from these objectives.[21] Also, they have selected students who have graduated from a health professional program or have had other training, have had a chance to see the world of practice, and have chosen to become qualified in a specific area.

In examining which of the variables might be manipulated reasonably readily in the model predicting geographic location of physicians, it should be noted that the kinds of physicians coming to training can be altered only via changes in medical education. The technical requirements related to practice and organizational requirements cannot be altered, and furthermore, the regulation of the resources of any one geographic area are well beyond the current state of the art of economics. The only independent variable that could be influenced is the numbers and types of sites for postgraduate training which would require, as indicated by Fein, coordinated action or else imposed federally determined decisions regarding how many of what kinds of specialties would be trained where.[22]

The rather depressing nature of all of the previous discussion leads me to suggest that *perhaps* existing institutions for the preparation of physicians *cannot* be altered significantly. Perhaps existing institutions producing specialists should be permitted and expected to do just that, and only that. If so, the output of these programs would need to be limited by controlling their numbers and by specifically determined federal support of postgraduate medical education for subspecialty and specialty practice. In the process we should also separate out government support of research, not to allocate it to "other" institutions (rather to the same institutions concerned with specialty training) but to be perfectly honest in what we are buying—research, cardiologists, thoracic surgeons, urologists, and so on.

A significant amount of the funds now supporting medical education/research/administration/service might be diverted to the support of other (new) institutions designed primarily to produce primary care providers. Since you can only spend it once, it will be necessary to divide the resources for the education of physicians and medical research into specific categories. I suggest the support of "other" or new institutions reflecting my belief that only when role models, curriculum structure, and institutional values, as well as the characteristics of students admitted can be significantly altered (and congruent), will we produce primary care practitioners in the number required. Some of these "institutions" might be existing medical schools, others might be programs preparing intermediate health workers such as physicians' assistants or nurse practitioners.

While the proposal to establish "separate and equal" medical schools to generate primary care physicians may have some appeal to certain groups, perhaps the major advantage of this suggestion is the value of such a threat to existing medical schools. Many believe that medical schools *are* capable of adaptation, providing the stimulus is of sufficient magnitude. Perhaps the creation of a specific time limit for the initiation of efforts to produce a significant proportion of primary care physicians will be necessary before established curriculum committees and other vested interests are willing to share some of their "power." The negative consequences of segregating programs developing primary care practitioners from existing educational institutions vastly outweigh potential advantages that might be created by generating a "pure culture" of primary care doctors. The process of separation would tend to insure their "uniqueness," and the problems of integrating primary, secondary, and tertiary levels of care, and the providers engaged in what should be a natural continuum of activities, would increase tremendously. In short, primary care physicians *must be* generated by existing medical schools even though the evidence would suggest that rather strenuous mandates from the federal government and private foundations will be necessary to accomplish the changes required to achieve this goal.

All of the preceding discussion has been directed at the solution of access to primary care physicians *wherever* they may be, for none of these changes will of necessity solve problems of access related to the geographic distribution of primary care providers. Some believe that programs preparing intermediate health workers such as physicians' assistants or nurse practitioners would provide the manpower for rural communities and inner-city areas. There is no reason to believe that these practitioners, who after all practice interdependently with physicians, will have any more enthusiasm for practicing in what might be described "undesirable" (to some) areas of the United States. In fact, in a Survey of Innovative Changes in Health Services that we have just completed, it has been somewhat depressing (although supportive of this contention) to find physicians' assistants located in rural communities planning to move back to the city. The problem has *not* been the acceptance of patients or support of the physician with whom they are working; in all cases it has been related to the fact their wives do not care to live in small communities.

ALLIED HEALTH PROFESSIONS AND TEAM CARE

I have not discussed two other means of increasing access to primary care. These include expansion of the numbers of allied health professionals and the functions and orientations of health teams.

The proliferation of "allied health professionals," that is, the generation of occupational therapists, radiologic technologists, and others, represents the consequences of a rapid expansion of knowledge, translated into action. The further differentiation within each of these areas into various levels, such as occupational therapy associates and occupational therapy aides, I believe, represents the natural history of professionalism. By this, I mean the tendency of any group, once defined as practicing a profession based upon scientific principles, as its membership increases to "define" further the scientific basis for its practice, to enlarge the requirements for certification in that field, thus staking off its "territory" more effectively, and finally to reach the point where there is a need to pass on certain tasks or functions previously performed by that group to a group of aides or associates prepared at a lower level. Society thus gains the benefit of more expert application of new knowledge and skills, but also acquires an economic burden related to fragmentation and inappropriate utilization of manpower. Allied health professionals, under these teams, provide services that complement and supplement those of the "primary health care provider," but none is seen as a potential replacement for the physician in his role of controlling access to all health care services.

Rhetoric about the "health care team" has diminished somewhat from the high level existing in the 1960s. I personally believe the concept of the health care team, while symbolically appealing to a variety of individuals, was most heartily endorsed by the physician because of the implications of his "captaincy" of that team. This approach provides a means of controlling the extent to which health services are provided by others and also avoids defaulting the game because of the absence of primary care providers to play the role of captain. It should be obvious from previous discussions that current medical education (as well as other health professional education) in no way prepares its future graduates to operate as "teams."

Before endorsing "team care" it is necessary to further define this concept. The first step is to distinguish among the several kinds of "teams" that exist in different settings, and the relative operational and functional nature of these arrangements. There are *intra*disciplinary teams—radiologist, surgeon, oncologist (all physicians)—that care for patients with malignant diseases. If one adds to that group specialized nursing care, social workers, occupational therapists and others, one has an *inter*disciplinary team, although its activities are relatively "simple" since all members of the group are concerned with the provision of care to patients with a specific disease/problem.

The type of "team" that functions in the operating room with hierarchical structure and clear division of functions, is obviously quite different from a "team" composed of psychiatrist, social worker, and occupational therapist who deal with disturbed children. The nature of the problems to be cared for suggest the components of a team and also the relative roles played by each member. A "team" composed of professionals from the several different disciplines needed to provide comprehensive services to chronically ill patients with multiple diseases/problems presents a real challenge to the "players."

In summary, the possibilities for solving the problem of access to primary care through minor alterations in the education of health professionals seem limited. Short of more radical changes, I can only conclude that the problems now under discussion will continue to become worse.

This somewhat dismal-cynical-realistic view emphasizes the need for alternative strategies to improve access to primary care, specifically those involving consumers.

CONSUMER EDUCATION

Consumers may be "taught" to use a system more effectively if there is something to be gained by them as a result of this effort on their part. What do consumers want and expect of health care services? Studies we have conducted among a variety of groups in Los Angeles including women's club members, young people, patients in a variety of settings, testify to the importance of access to care, specifically to emergency services. We have asked several hundred individuals to rank in order of preference a variety of types of health care services including seeing the same doctor each visit, access to emergency care on a 24-hour basis, relief from pain, services that will detect disease at an early stage and so on. Among all social and ethnic groups independent of sex and past history of medical problems, consumers are most concerned with the availability of emergency care 24 hours a day and the immediate relief of pain. Compared to these two, all other aspects of care seem less important.

These two needs are met in a single type of facility—the emergency room/area/department. The disappearance of primary care providers or physicians who will take new patients is reflected in the numbers of visits to "emergency rooms" for nonemergent problems, at least as defined by the physician. As visits to emergency facilities have increased, additional problems have been generated for those concerned with the operation of these facilities. A significant number of true medical emergencies arrive intermixed with "primary care problems" and these two streams must be triaged or separated. The "emergency room" has become for many communities the only sure access to primary care. Significant organizational and administrative problems have been created by this trend, and we are still in the early stages of experimenting with solutions to these problems.

While adult consumers of care may be given a course in "how to win in the clinics," I doubt that this is a viable or cost-effective solution since if they find it possible to "beat the system" in large numbers, the system may change in order to avoid dealing with them.

Perhaps a more significant and long-term solution could be achieved through the *development* of more appropriate consumer decision-making. There are adequate data to document the extent of inappropriate utilization of health services by adults. A significant number of individuals delay in the face of warning signs and symptoms of serious disease[23]; a majority of individuals fail to comply with physicians' recommendations for treatment of their medical problems[24, 25]; only a few individuals asked to return for routine preventive screening examinations, do so[26]; from 12 percent to 15 percent of adults in any health services program utilize 40 to 50 percent of all health services available.[27]

While there have been several studies attempting to explain the utilization of health care services by adults, only a minor part of the variation has been explained.[28] In contrast, there have been few studies of the *origins* of health attitudes, beliefs, and behaviors. As a result of some incidental observations made during the late 1960s, we became interested in the determinants of health and illness behavior in young children, and the natural history of these phenomena. We are currently finishing a two-year preliminary study concerned with the interrelations of social, psychological, and developmental variables as they influence young children's perceptions of what is illness and what are appropriate reasons for seeking care. The second year of our study has been directed at an experimental intervention labeled "Child-Initiated Pediatric Care."[29] In this research we have utilized an experimental elementary school and staffed the health service with pediatric nurse practitioners. We have created an adult-free "care system" that permits children to seek care directly from a nurse practitioner whenever they (the children) feel so inclined. We have structured the interactions between nurse practitioner-child so that the child is placed in a decision-making role. For example, the child is asked what his problem is, what he thinks might be wrong. He is examined by the nurse who provides feedback of appropriate data ("your temperature is normal, you don't have any signs of infection in your ears or throat"); he is asked what he thinks ought to be done. Children are given a variety of options (within permissible limits) for their own self-disposition. Whenever "appropriate" decisions are made ("I guess I'll go back to class"), these are reinforced by the nurse practitioner; children making inappropriate decisions are allowed to do so, but as evidence accumulates these children have been identified and attempts are made to alter this pattern of decision-making.

The study might be considered to be an approach to the creation of a socialization mechanism for the development of responsible utilizers of health services through active involvement as consumer-decision-makers. The results are very fragmentary at this stage and all I can report is that the findings with regard to children's perceptions of health, causes of illness, and reasons for seeking care, are consistent with current theories of child development. We have also noticed in our initial studies the importance of "access" to care for children. Early in the research, when asking about the availability of school nurse services, we were struck by the fact that some children, particularly those from disadvantaged areas, indicated they could not get to see the nurse. This occurred in schools where there was considerable, although not *complete,* nursing coverage. In the experimental study we have provided service coverage for every hour that school was in session during the week, to avoid generating the impression that the nurse was not "accessible." All that seems necessary to create the impression of non-accessibility is to have a child show up at the nurse's office at any random point in time and find the room empty.

Unless we are able somehow to alter the development of current adult behavior patterns related to the utilization of health services, perhaps other proposed solutions to improve access may have little meaning.

SELF-HELP OR LET ME DO IT

The provision of health services by the consumer himself is not new. Those of you who have examined any of the books commonly available at the turn of the 20th century appreciate that, once again, health services are rediscovering the past.[30] The contention in the early 1900s that individuals should know enough about common problems to be able to take care of themselves in the absence of a physician was based upon a problem of access. The self-help movement, in some instances, is confounded with women's rights, or the needs of groups with certain social or ideological characteristics to reject the physician and to be independent of the chauvinistic, authoritarian, manipulative individuals who exercise considerable control over their bodies and "rights." The hazards of self-help in 1973 are somewhat greater than in 1900, due to the number of potent drugs available for the "treatment" of disease. While there may be some risk involved, perhaps self-help in one form or another may be the *only* answer to the problem of access to primary care for those in isolated or rural communities throughout the United States.

Within the past two or three years there has been increased effort in the development and testing of so-called "protocols" for the management of medical problems by relatively unskilled providers.[31] These protocols have been used by physicians' assistants in certain programs.[32] We are using them, not as a guide for the management of patients by nurse practitioners, but as a form of programmed instruction in the UCLA Primex program. A protocol should reflect the distilled essence of "clinical judgment," utilizing what is known about the relative importance of certain signs, symptoms, and laboratory findings in the differential diagnosis or classification of a patient with a complaint such as sore throat or headache, into a specific diagnostic entity. There is evidence this approach is feasible. The key questions that remain unanswered are what are the specific problems-complaints that are susceptible to the "protocol" approach, and what level of preparation is required for the utilization of different kinds of protocols. Some require a background usually attributable to a graduate nurse; others can be utilized by "high school graduates." We are now preparing to test a variety of these protocols on consumers to determine the extent to which they might be fashioned into a self-help curriculum.

The selection of local "citizens" interested in health services and their training in the use of protocols might be considered to be equivalent to generating barefoot doctors carrying cookbooks for care. However, this approach, coupled with the requisite backup communication links—not an improbability given the technological sophistication of the United States—may be the only means of providing access to care for a significant portion of our population. Such an approach means accepting the probability that we will *never* generate a sufficient number of primary care physicians, or intermediate health practitioners so that remote or "unpopular" areas of the United States will have an adequate supply of "trained" health manpower.

PREVENTIVE MEDICINE

Certainly the ultimate solution to the problems of access to care would be to prevent the need for requiring access. However, since a great number of primary care problems are not solely biological in origin, but have considerable psychosocial components, this means not only preventing disease, but also dealing with behaviors associated with the causes of disease. The primary causes of many diseases in the United States have their roots in the life style of our citizens. To date, there is little evidence that behavioral modification mechanisms have sufficiently persuaded individuals to alter their patterns of living, i.e., to discontinue smoking, increase exercise, reduce their weight, etc. Preventive medicine practices that are not based upon altering the biological composition of the patient would seem to have limited success in the immediate future.

SUMMARY

As indicated, the word "reform," which is part of the title, has a variety of meanings such as (1) to change from bad to good, (2) to restore to former goodness, (3) to change for the better by alteration. All of these imply value judgments—we must ask what is "good"? defined by whom? access to whom for what?

In 1973 most medical educators would say that the American people have never had it so good. I suspect most practitioners of medicine would respond similarly. Apparently a significant proportion of consumers do not believe that the present status of health services is "optimal" or "good," but again, "compared to what?" "Goodness" cannot imply the reversal of social change. A great deal has happened in American society since 1940. Values have changed. A variety of the changes that would improve access to care through educational means might be seen as decreasing the freedom of individual choice, both for providers and consumers. Whether or not society as a whole considers it "good" to decrease the options available to those seeking to become physicians and to increase the responsibility of patients through behavior modification, forced alteration of life style, or other means, may well determine future patterns of health care in the United States.

REFERENCES

1. Ingersoll, R. W. and Graves, G. O., Predictability of Success in the First Year of Medical School, *Journal of Medical Education*, 40, 351-63, 1965.

2. Coker, R. E., Jr., Medical Careers and Public Health, *Milbank Memorial Fund Quarterly*, 44, 181-228, 1966.

3. Lewis, C. E. and Easton, R. E., Personality Characteristics, Career Interests, Observed Health Behavior and the Teaching of Community Medicine, *Archives of Environmental Health,* 21, 99-104, 1970.

4. Monk, M. A. and Thomas, C. B., Characteristics of Male Medical Students Related to Their Subsequent Careers, *Johns Hopkins Medical Journal,* 127, 254-72, 1970.

5. Schumacher, C. F., Personal Characteristics of Students Choosing Different Types of Medical Careers, *Journal of Medical Education,* 39, 278-88, 1964.

6. Lewis, C. E., A Longitudinal Study of Potential Change—Agents in Medicine— A Preliminary Report, *Journal of Medical Education,* 44, 1029-34, 1969.

7. Schofield, W., Research Studies of Medical Students and Physicians Utilizing Standard Personality Instruments: An Annotated Bibliography, Association of American Medical Colleges, 52 pages, 1972.

8. Lewis, C. E., Use of Preventive Medicine Case Summaries: Analysis of 1400 Reports, *Archives of Environmental Health,* 14, 889-903, 1967.

9. Lewis, C. E., Unpublished data.

10. Lewis, C. E. and Resnick, B., Relative Orientations of Students of Medicine and Nursing in Ambulatory Patient Care, *Journal of Medical Education,* 41, 162-66, 1966.

11. Sloan, F. A., Lifetime Earnings and Physicians' Choice of Specialty, *Industrial and Labor Relations Review,* 24, 47-56, 1970.

12. Lewis, C. E. and Arnold, M. A., The Professional Wife (In press).

13. Miller, G., TEACHING AND LEARNING IN MEDICAL SCHOOL, Harvard University Press, Cambridge, Massachusetts, 1961, p. 304.

14. Clifford, M. and Walster, E., The Effect of Physical Attractiveness, *Sociology of Education,* 46, 248-58, 1973.

15. Rosenthal, R. and Jacobson, L., PYGMALION IN THE CLASSROOM, Holt, Rinehart and Winston, New York, 1968.

16. Fein, R. and Weber, G., FINANCING MEDICAL EDUCATION: AN ANALYSIS OF ALTERNATIVE POLICIES AND MECHANISMS, McGraw-Hill, New York, 1971.

17. Butter, I., The Migratory Flow of Doctors To and From University States, *Medical Care*, 9, 17-31, 1971.

18. Joroff, S. and Navarro, V., Medical Manpower: A Multivariate Analysis of the Distribution of Physicians in Urban United States, *Medical Care*, 9, 429-38, 1971.

19. Yett, D. and Sloan, F., Analysis of Migration Patterns of Recent Medical Graduates (Mimeo). Presented at Health Services Research Conference on Factors in Health Manpower Performance and the Delivery of Health Care, Chicago, Dec. 9, 1971.

20. Lewis, C. E. and Shonick, W., Determinants of the Distribution of Kansas Physicians (In press).

21. Lewis, C. E., Evaluation of the Performance of Intermediate Health Workers. Presented at the Macy Conference on Intermediate Health Manpower, Williamsburg, Virginia, 13-14 Nov. 1972.

22. Fein, R., On Achieving Access and Equity in Health Care, in Andreopoulos, S. (Editor), MEDICAL CURE AND MEDICAL CARE, *Milbank Memorial Fund Quarterly*, 50, 157-90, 1972, Part 2.

23. Kasl, S. V. and Cobb, S., Some Psychological Factors Associated with Illness Behavior and Selected Illnesses, *Journal of Chronic Diseases*, 17, 325-45, 1964.

24. Davis, M. S., Predicting Non-Compliant Behavior, *Journal of Health and Social Behavior*, 8, 265-71, 1967.

25. Bergman, A. B. and Werner, R. J., Failure of Children to Receive Penicillin by Mouth, *New England Journal of Medicine*, 268, 1334-38, 1963.

26. Lewis, C. E., Consumer Control of Carcinoma of the Cervix (In press).

27. Avnet, H. H., PHYSICIAN SERVICE PATTERNS AND ILLNESS RATES, Group Health Insurance, Inc., New York, 1967, p. 451.

28. Battistella, R. M., Limitations in Use of the Concept of Psychological Readiness to Initiate Health Care, *Medical Care*, 6, 308-18, 1968.

29. Lewis, C. E. and Lewis, M. A., Child Initiated Pediatric Care, Research in progress, UCLA, 1971-73.

30. Fallos, R. and Truitt, B., KNOW THYSELF, S. A. Mullikan, Marietta, Ohio, 1911.

31. Blackburn, J., Bragg, F. E., Greenfield, S. and McCraith, D. L., Protocol for Upper Respiratory Complaints, Project Report ACP-25, Lincoln Laboratory and Beth Israel Hospital, M.I.T., Cambridge, Massachusetts, 1972.

32. Sox, H. C., Jr., Sox, C. H. and Tompkins, R. K., Training of Physicians' Assistants by a Clinical Algorithm System, *New England Journal of Medicine,* 288, 818-23, 1973.

II THE EVOLUTION OF A

PRIMARY CARE SYSTEM

CHAPTER 3 • STANLEY S. BERGEN, JR.

Primary Health Care: Suggested Organizational Structure

A few months ago, as I drove along one of the main streets of the city in which I live, a street that has traditionally been populated by the private offices of practicing physicians within the community, I noted a hand-lettered sign nailed to a tree. It read: *Primary Medicine Physicians.* My first reaction was that this sign had been prepared by children or teenagers as an advertisement for a Health Fair or a similar event. On closer examination, I realized that the sign in fact designated a physician's office where three practicing physicians had joined to practice what they had chosen to identify as "Primary Medicine."

About two weeks after this event, while attending a luncheon to initiate the Community Fund Campaign in a large urban community, I entered into conversation with a group of the attendees as they discussed the practice of medicine in their neighborhoods. One woman volunteered with great pride that she had recently had the good fortune to be referred to a "primary physician." She hastened to tell all those who were listening that this physician was one who took care of the medical needs of her "entire family," with particular attention to the "routine illnesses that no other doctor seems to want to care for today." Many of the others in the group looked upon this lady with great envy. You could see the anxieties in their faces and the amazement in her good fortune in being able to contact and, in fact, secure the services of a physician who would care for and be available to her entire family. I believe these two separate, yet in a strange way connected events, indicate a significant change in the attitude of the public concerning medical care.

We hear many claims of the crisis in American medicine, the health care crisis and dramatic examples of individuals and families unable to secure adequate health care. The real crisis, if that is indeed the correct descriptive term, is not one of quality or expertise but rather one of access. We are all aware of the great strides made in the medical sciences during the last 30 years and the

101

benefits that have been provided for many of the American public by these advances and the specialization of our physicians. I do not believe that any of us would wish to sacrifice the success of the medical profession or its educational process nor would we wish to place ourselves in the hands of less qualified practitioners when we are acutely ill, when a complicated disease process has defied diagnosis or when a particular diagnosis has indicated the need of a specialist for its treatment. Engle[1] has warned against abandoning the beneficial attainments of our current medical education and training programs as we attempt to find new solutions to correct a failing delivery system. Annis[2] recently urged modification and improvement in the delivery system through increased training programs for primary physicians and better distribution of such physicians to all segments of the population. Peterson[3] has called dramatic attention to the serious defect in our current system noting the apparent excess of neurosurgeons in practice in New England compared to the number in England. Since England does not seem to suffer from the lack of adequate neurosurgery expertise, this may be an example of the health system actually creating illness. Bergland[4] feels the motivation for the training of neurosurgeons may be more one of training program requirements rather than service needs. Many of the public have gradually and conclusively become aware of the lack of an accessible entry point for medical care.

Many times each week I am asked by a friend, a visitor or a casual caller for the name of a physician to care for their family: "You know, doctor, someone who can see us quickly when the children are sick and yet take care of my husband and me at the same time" or "a doctor like my family had when I was a child." It may be a myth but the public perception of the family physician or the general practitioner is one of a readily available professional who will make home visits, render general acute care combined with a long-term interest, compassion and knowledge of family problems and health. One of the most forceful pressures for change in the health care delivery system is the feeling by the public of a lack of access to primary care and an identifiable entry point to a physician who can act not only as healer but confidante and counselor. The large expenditures of both private and public funds for various aspects of health care rightfully have led the consumers to believe that such a system should be more responsive to needs both real and perceived. At a time when over $80 billion or in excess of 7 percent of the gross national product is allocated for expenditures relating to all health care activities, and when we look forward to 1980 and a possible dedication of as much as 9.8 percent of the GNP[5] to health, it is not unreasonable for the public to expect such resources to be directed toward development of a system of health care that will provide primary care services for a larger segment of the population now served. Peterson[3] has recently noted that Great Britain uses 5.5 percent of its GNP for health services and yet access to general medical care has not seemed to be a problem in that nation.

In considering the organizational changes that might provide access to a source of primary care and an organizational structure that might be developed to provide such care, a series of questions must be posed:

1. Has the hospital become an appropriate source of primary care?
2. Should new and different health care personnel be utilized to render primary care and/or should more physicians be educated to provide primary care?
3. If other than physicians are utilized, how should they be regulated and would they be part of a group effort or act as independent practitioners?
4. Should a new type of physician be educated to staff the new organizational system?
5. Should an entirely new system be developed or can we build on existing resources?
6. Will group practice, HMO's, prepay capitation and medical care foundations improve access and have an impact on the availability of primary care?

For purposes of this discussion the following definitions will be used to identify the components of health care to be involved:

Primary medicine is the practice of initial contact health care, provided in a continuous manner to patients following development of a comprehensive plan of health maintenance that takes cognizance of the patient's clinical, social, psychological, behavioral and community needs. While a single individual assumes responsibility for each patient and/or the family unit, a group of professionals may join in the provision of various components of primary health care.

Primary physician is the physician approached by individuals or family units seeking medical advice and treatment on a continuing basis, personal care, preventive care and health maintenance. He may or may not function as a member of a team of providers in various practice settings.

Family physician is the physician of initial contact who acts as the entry point into the health care system, evaluates his patient's total health needs, provides personal care within his competence and refers to appropriate specialists or community agencies as necessary while acting as coordinator of the patient's spectrum of health services. He may or may not function as a member of a team of providers in various practice settings.

THE PROBLEM: APPROACHES TO A SOLUTION

Never before has it been more necessary for the country to develop a national policy on health[6] and medical education.[7] Before critical decisions are made concerning the form and structure of national entitlement, a consensus of national philosophy must be determined. As we approach the creation of such policy the problem of access to primary care and primary care facilities for all consumers, the urban poor, the suburban middle class and the rural population, will become a major challenge. Among others, three paths could be chosen to improve access to primary care:

Increased numbers of physicians could be made available to the system and thus to patients

The ultimate goal of such an effort would be to provide enough physicians so that the mechanisms of economics would force many of the additional physicians to distribute themselves more evenly geographically and by discipline to all segments of the population. Unfortunately there can be no assurance that this would in fact result since we note from past experience that most physicians tend to gravitate to those areas of access to hospital facilities, better living conditions for their families and areas attractive to their practice which has been increasingly specialty oriented. The development of a special category of physicians such as suggested by Proger,[8] whereby some physicians would be trained to deliver primary care, might easily lead to the further development of a two-class system. All physicians should receive equal quality training, and through the process of preselection during admission[9] or through a natural phenomena society, the pattern of change[10] would be directed so that young physicians could be attracted into the disciplines of primary care.

In 1931, 80 percent of the practicing physicians in the United States considered themselves general practitioners. In 1970 this figure had fallen to 21 percent with an additional 14 percent of pediatricians and internists considering themselves as delivering primary care.[11] Much of this change was dictated by social pressures following World War II which demanded increased research in biomedical science, with emphasis upon the improvement of the treatment of disease. This tremendous interest was accompanied by large federal subsidy programs that influenced the medical schools and thus their products, the medical students and young physicians, into specialty practice and research. Concomitantly, the increase in instrumentation within our hospitals and the development of hospitals as specialty care institutions attracted young physicians into this mode of practice.

Today we see definite evidence of a trend in the opposite direction. While some western countries such as Canada continue to consider over 50 percent of their practicing physicians as general practitioners or family physicians,[12] only recently has the trend to specialty practice begun to reverse in the United States. In 1970, 3 percent of physicians in training (internships and residencies) were in areas of general practice. However in 1972 there were 133 approved residencies in family practice, 77 located in community hospitals, 48 at university affiliated hospitals, and 8 in the Armed Forces. As of July 1, 1972, there were 470 first-year residents training in family practice; there were 350 in the second year, and 189 in the third year—a total of 1009 in training.

A total of 105 medical schools were surveyed as of July, 1972. Of these, 34 had departments of family practice, and 31 had divisions of family practice, 14 of which were free standing and 17 located in other departments of instruction. Nineteen other departments of family practice are under development by medical schools. In 1969 there were 30 programs for the training of family practitioners. In 1972 the number rose to 133 with a projection of up to 207 family practice training programs[13] through 1975. A recent report by Herrmann[14] notes there has been a major shift of interest toward primary care training by graduates of the University of Michigan Medical School in 1971 and 1972, with 33 and 61.7 percent matching in the respective years studied. There were 1050 family practice residencies offered in 1973 with 1600 planned for 1975.* Since such indicators are good measures of supply and demand we should not move toward separate medical school educational processes for family practitioners or primary physicians, but rather continue to stimulate our young students and physicians to move toward the concept of comprehensive primary care.

THE DEVELOPMENT OF DIFFERENT TYPES OF HEALTH CARE DELIVERY PERSONNEL

For years many countries have utilized trained persons other than physicians to deliver primary health care services to patients. The use of the *Feldsher* in Russia[15] has been well described and well known. The use of public health nurses, physician assistants or support personnel in other locations is also adequately documented.[16,17] In the United States over the last few years, we have seen a burgeoning interest in the utilization of physician assistants.[18] The development of the Duke physicians' assistants program in the early 1960s,[19] the MEDEX program in Washington[20] and similar programs, directed both toward primary care and specialty services, has been reported and reviewed. In addition the development of pediatric nurse practitioners in Colorado[21] and use of other types of health care personnel, such as family health workers, mental health case aides, etc., has proven that nonphysicians, particularly those specifically task oriented, can deliver personal health services to patients in need. The sole responsibility for the delivery of primary health care should not be vested in such personnel, but rather the functions of such disciplines should be with practicing primary health care physicians or family practitioners who can, through a team effort, address the primary care needs of our population. To utilize allied health personnel as sole practitioners to expand our primary health care system, would merely provide an additional parameter to our present dual system of health care—a system that pits private against public facilities, inpatient facilities against outpatient facilities and the specialist against the generalist. Such a continued trend would be divisive.

---

*According to latest figures published in the September 1973 issue of *Medical World News*, three-year family residency programs have climbed much faster than these earlier projections. As of July, 1973, there were 755 residents in the first year, 654 in the second year, and 354 in the third year—a total of 1,754 in training. There are currently 145 family practice training programs in operation, 29 more with approval but not yet operating and about 20 with approval pending.—*Editor*.

DEVELOPMENT OF AN ACCESSIBLE
PRIMARY HEALTH CARE DELIVERY SYSTEM

The development of a primary health care delivery system must be attractive to the patient and to the physician. The patient must be attracted to a system he finds accessible and within his ability for cost, convenience and sensitivity to his needs. There is no doubt a pluralistic system will and should continue in the United States. As noted by Somers,[22] this system cannot be sacrificed nor should it be sacrificed for a totally new care delivery system. Rather, we must change, improve and reorganize the existing system in a manner to improve its accessibility and delivery potential.

The first two methods of improving access to primary health care will be left to other authors for their review and suggestions. The use and availability of additional physicians and other health care personnel will be mentioned only tangently as they refer to the development of a system for primary health care delivery and its administrative and organizational structure and relationships.

If one attempts to change a delivery system to provide greater access to primary health care, one must be sure there is in fact a need for such service. Other than the emotional interest noted by individuals and families, is there any proof that in fact we do not have sufficiently available primary health care facilities or primary care delivery personnel at this time?

A study conducted over 10 years ago revealed that out of 1,000 patients, 750 will have one or more illnesses during any month; 250 of these individuals will consult a physician, 9 will be admitted to a hospital, 5 will be referred to other physicians and 1 will be admitted to a university medical center.[23] Thus, we can see that for 25 percent of the population there is an apparent need for some type of medical care each month. However, only 1.5 percent of those at risk require either hospital admission or referral to a specialist for more intensive care. Therefore, over 98 percent of the population seeking health care during a month are seeking this attention for episodes of illness that seems to be of a primary health care nature. These could be and should be handled by health care personnel, oriented toward primary medical problems.

Using these statistics, one cannot predict the effect of preventive medicine nor can one determine how many of these episodes will require follow-up visits for continuous medical care. One can only surmise that a continuous relationship with a physician or health team would create an atmosphere of continuity of care in a manner oriented toward the entire family as a medical and social unit and that such orientation could possibly further reduce the need for inpatient and/or specialist care.

A recent article by Gandevia[10] relates the history of the evolution of general practice in Australia. He notes that the first practitioners were required to adapt to the terrain, the social needs of the early settlers and the isolation that was imposed by the long distances between the settlements. He notes also that the question "was not which physician, but the physician." Gandevia[10] observes that the characteristics of the population and their social demands dictated the practice of the physicians. Being relatively young and healthy, the population was not particularly prone to chronic or degenerate disease, except for those who had sought out Australia as a possible site for improvement of various lung conditions. The services of a physician were required to care for a wide spectrum of acute trauma and illness. As townships began to develop, specialists were required to man the hospitals created to serve the larger collections of the population. A general practitioner soon learned that economic remuneration as a specialist was increased and that his status as a physician was enhanced. With the increased scientific approach to medicine in the last 25 years, the author notes a trend toward greater specialization. However in recent years, society has once again made demands for the need for primary care. The profession has begun to adapt itself by attempting to restore a satisfying general practice or family practice mode of health care. Gandevia is convinced that society, not the profession, will dictate the needs and pattern of care of the future as it has in the past.

At least three major reports of commissioned groups or an individual,[24-26] in the mid-1960s, called for the development of primary care facilities and the education of increased numbers of primary health care personnel. Studies of utilization patterns of general practitioners,[27] urban,[28] small town,[29] and rural physicians,[30] have all indicated a preponderance of primary health care needs and the increasing tendency to rely on health teams and hospital emergency rooms to provide such care. As this evolution has occurred, teaching hospitals have and must continue to assume greater responsibility for comprehensive care services for the local population.[31-32]

Hospital emergency rooms[33] have played an increasing role in the provision of primary health care services over the last few years not only for the medically indigent but also for referrals from private practitioners. Fifty percent of such patients do not need emergency care, 33 percent have no other source of primary care, 33 percent consider the emergency room their usual source of health care and about 20 percent require emergency care or hospitalization.[34-35] Emergency rooms can carry out the responsibility of triage, evaluation and placing priority upon the needs of individual patients. Referrals from the emergency room should be made to primary care facilities, inpatient facilities or specialists as necessary, with emphasis placed upon referrals to primary care facilities to assure the initiation of ongoing comprehensive care for each individual patient. The critical defects of both the outpatient and emergency room system of primary health care as they function currently are inadequate patient follow-up and inadequate professional communications concerning patients' conditions.[36]

Fisher[37] studied 150 patients chosen at random during a five-week period from the University of Oklahoma Hospital outpatient department. All patients were seeking care or advice concerning problems that normally would be dealt with by a family physician or a primary care physician. Patient response was most favorable toward physicians functioning in an outpatient medical clinic, who took the greatest amount of time and showed the greatest interest in the patients' complaints. Patients tended to consider a physician's care good if he explained the nature of their illness and/or disability. Dissatisfaction was expressed in the lack of continuity of care, failing to see the same physician on repeat visits, long waiting time and negative reactions based on previous poor experience with such outpatient medical care.

A similar study recently appeared in the *Annals of Internal Medicine.* [38] The study reviewed the experience of 116 patients with gastrointestinal symptoms who presented at the emergency room at the Johns Hopkins Hospital. Results revealed that 25 percent received satisfactory care and an additional 14 percent received adequate treatment. Added to the questionable quality and satisfaction is the oft-noted fragmentation both of professional service and administrative functions[39] in such facilities.

Clearly there is a need for an improved system for the delivery of primary health care and a demand for such care.

Beloff, Weinerman *et al.*[40-41] felt that the Family Health Care Project at Yale had produced improved comprehensive medical care with emphasis placed upon the health maintenance of families. They felt that such care must be highly organized before delivery can be contemplated and that the team approach is the most feasible for such organized care. Team conferences, unit records, fact sheets, log and utilization data are all important components of such care.

Proger[8] has urged the elimination of the omnicompetent concept of the single physician's ability to deliver the total spectrum of health care. Many have urged consideration of the team to provide for health care delivery needs.[36, 41-45]. A strong central unified professional and administrative authority has been suggested by some authors,[46-48] while others have indicated a desire for greater decentralization.[42] Primary health care should be directed toward evaluation of the whole patient with specific attention to current problems. Referrals should be made to specialists for consultation only with the return of the patient to the primary care physician to assure continuity and a continued relationship between them. Medical control is necessary to direct patients to whom to go to receive appropriate care for the situation.

Peterson,[27] discussing the primary physician as a "high productivity physician," feels that one of the problems facing us today is the need to clarify the functions and training of the "ideal core physician or primary practitioner," what has been referred to as "the practice of personal medicine."[49] As noted above there is no lack of interest among current medical students toward entering such careers provided the system is made more rewarding professionally and organizationally.

A recent study conducted at five medical schools in England[50] concerned the attitudes of medical students toward general practice. The survey revealed that students questioned in the first, third and fifth years are more favorably disposed toward general practice during their educational careers. These students felt that it is unfair and incorrect that the general practitioners are prevented from access to the hospital to care for their patients and to become aware of scientific advancement. The favorable trend toward primary care careers seems to indicate a desire for more direct contact with patients as people. The British students expressed their feeling that the greatest difficulty facing general practice was that of "keeping up" with current developments in the practice of medicine. They felt that medical schools should orient themselves more toward teaching students better patient relations and patterns of care in a more organized system. They felt that exposure in medical school had a direct relationship to the career choices made by students. Garrison,[51] writing in the *Journal of the American Geriatric Society* in 1971 noted that the inadequate supply of family or front line physicians must be related to the lack of access for these physicians to appropriate health care facilities. At that time, he noted that government and society had not made the same contributions to the education or practice of family physicians that they have to specialists. Facilities, financial assistance in training programs and equipment have been provided for specialists. Family medicine programs and medical schools require similar support for educational activities and research potential in primary care. Financing from the government should provide special incentives for those entering the area of family practice, particularly for those entering urban areas. Millar[52] has noted that much of primary medical care is involved in the unrewarding, unsatisfying and insoluble time wasting activities of caring for the well or the near well. He felt that the use of paramedical personnel in these areas should not be to the exclusion of the physician but as part of a team. Millar[52] urged that the physician not be made into a social agency but rather included in the overall health care delivery system, giving the general practitioner or family physician access to the hospital. He noted that although allied health personnel can be of great assistance in the delivery of primary care, they cannot fulfill the role of the physician without being taught diagnosis and then they may as well be developed into physicians. He felt that the current system of primary care led to the development of a family physician by education and then denied him use of his knowledge by keeping him away from the hospital, the hospital environment and an organized system. Gilbert,[53] writing in the *Canadian Medical Association Journal* has noted that the primary physician has a unique role. However, he felt that this role must be more clearly defined and that it must be decided who will deliver primary health care. An editorial in *Lancet*[42] has noted the conflicts of role and status which have brought continuing change to the need for an interest in general practice or primary care. The author urged the small hospital as the base for primary health care delivery much as Analyn[54] had suggested that such activities be under the control of consumer-provider "area health boards"[42] to provide for structure and proper allocation of resources. The continued attraction of primary care will depend on the development of an organizational system that will equalize access for all physicians to all components of the health care delivery system. Physicians can no longer be sequestrated into ambulatory care facilities or away from access to hospitals.

Crawford[55] studied the reasons primary physicians left practice to seek other medical careers. The three most commonly noted reasons were: overwork, unsystematic approach to medical care and the lack of adequate available facilities. Also mentioned were the greater prestige in alternate career activities, controlled hours of work and increased access by specialists to facilities that would allow improved delivery of care. Crawford felt the attrition could be stopped by better organization of primary care administration and interpretation of the critical aspects of primary care through better educational opportunities in medical school and continuing education efforts.

The British Medical Association report on primary medical care[43] noted the need for greater organization of the system, particularly at ambulatory care units away from the hospital where groups of professionals could work as a team. The needs for hospital access, role and function clarification were also echoed in this report.

THE NEED FOR PRIMARY CARE

The needs for primary health care and personnel have been identified as have some of the prerequisites to viability. By placing emphasis on ambulatory care, economies can be realized by greater utilization of such facilities versus more costly inpatient beds.[56] Andrews[57] reported a 250 percent increase in ambulatory primary health care services in Sweden from 1952 to 1966 as greater organization and primary health care orientation was brought to the system. In the past the hospital has often provided ambulatory care as a mechanism to recruit inpatients and fulfill training program requirements.[58] As hospitals assume a greater role in the delivery of primary health care[32] they must stress ambulatory care functions both at the hospital and in off-site locations with equal funding and status accorded to such programs and staff. The hospital will then become the central focus for a "primary health care network," while continuing to fulfill the role as provider of specialty back-up consultative, laboratory and radiology services and inpatient facilities.

As such a system develops we must follow White's[6] direction and provide for public regulation and understanding of the health care delivery system. The needs of the consumer within this new more structured system will be served better if the orientation changes from one where the physician and hospital create a self-serving monopoly through sole decision-making authority "to one where society's needs are met through society's action."[6] One such mechanism of negotiated control might be the contract or franchise as suggested by Somers.[59]

All parts of the problem will not be adequately addressed or solutions found unless we develop a new organizational system that considers the need for primary health care as not merely the initial point of effort but one part of the whole. Analyn[54] has divided health care into various levels, designating locations and responsibilities for each level. He identifies individual personal hygiene and self-care as the initial level closely linked to buddy care or first aid. He designates a progression from triage emergency units, primary care hospitals and regional centers to academic health science centers with increasing levels of personnel expertise and sophistication of equipment. The local community hospital would be staffed by health care teams trained in the delivery of primary medical care. Such a team would include health workers, nurses, physician assistants and physicians. At the regional hospital and the university medical centers, specialists would be available accompanied by adequate facilities and personnel. Each element of the system would have a degree of independence from the others, although there must be continuity between the elements both for the transfer of information and for the continuity of care.

While accepting Analyn's[54] general concepts there must be consumer involvement in priority decision making, with physician and consumer access at all levels in such a regional network plan.

CATEGORICAL PROGRAMS

At present, some of our most successful primary health care delivery programs, particularly for the indigent, are directed toward categorical illnesses. Detection and prevention programs, such as maternal and infant care, family planning and communicable diseases, whether delivered by federal sponsorship or through state health departments, have been hallmarks in the delivery of primary health care to the consumer.[60] These programs have been successful and should be continued as part of a comprehensive health care program effort. Categorical programs fragment care no matter how effective in their own area. Mental health care, and the treatment and prevention of drug addiction and alcoholism should also be combined into a single program of primary health care. The further fragmentation of primary care services in the categorical programs will increase costs and continue to divide our health care delivery system into disease-oriented programs at the expense of health maintenance. Some categorical programs have attempted to approach their patients' primary needs by referrals to existing systems for further medical evaluation. Unfortunately this dependence on nonintegrated services has led to less than satisfactory results. At times, categorical programs can act as access to the system for primary health care and as a monitoring device for specific illnesses when detected. It must be recognized, however, that when financial rewards are oriented toward a single disease, categorical program staffs can only provide limited general care to patients with a broad spectrum of complaints.

COORDINATION OF EXISTING RESOURCES

Categorical programs in maternal and infant care, family planning, communicable diseases, joined with the programs for the treatment of alcoholism, drug addiction and mental health, could provide the basis for a general primary care medical program. Such a grouping of programs could be built into existing funding if a strong regulatory mechanism forcing a coordinated comprehensive package is included.

Utilizing existing hospitals as focal points for coordination, a regionalized system embracing existing categorical programs, outpatient departments, free-standing health centers, satellite clinics, group and solo practitioners could be combined into a primary health care system. With Medicaid and Medicare as a base, incremental increases in financial coverage could be developed toward full shared entitlement.

MEDICAL SCHOOL ROLE IN PRIMARY CARE DELIVERY

In recent years, medical and dental schools have, with increasing frequency, begun to play a role in the delivery of health care directly to patient populations.[61-62] Medical schools have come to realize that they need to assume a role in the delivery of personal health services through family health care units, and development of new health care delivery systems that would provide educational models for their students and house staff. It would seem that this potential should be examined in greater depth and that careful consideration should be given to the use of medical schools, where available, joining with their affiliated hospitals as a source for a regional health care delivery system for a geographic area or a population group.[63]

THE HOSPITAL: AMBULATORY CARE

Neighborhood family health centers could serve as a basic element in the creation of a primary health care system in urban areas,[64] while group practices and solo practitioners working with teams of allied health professionals could provide primary care in rural areas.[65] This would develop a total coverage system as outlined by Donabedian,[65] with the hospital and medical school providing the ultimate control center by delegating authority and responsibility to the smaller component units. This geographic distribution of care has been developed in other countries with apparent beneficial effects on the total health care and delivery system and improvement of accessibility for the consumers. An example of such a system has recently been reviewed by Andrews in his article on medical care in Sweden.[57] Current interests would dictate an examination of at least four possible structural units that might participate in an overall organization to deliver primary care to a geographic or regionalized area. These elements are health maintenance organizations, foundations for medical care, Neighborhood Health Centers and Hospital Ambulatory Care Units.

If we are to build upon the existing system and its strengths, hospital ambulatory care units must be considered as a potential building block. Relationships could be created between ambulatory care units and the inpatient services of hospitals both as back-up facilities and as recruiters of health care personnel to staff satellite units. At the same time, we must be aware that hospital ambulatory care units in the past have not risen to the challenge of providing care for patients in need nor have they provided this care as a primary thrust of the institution, but rather as a supplementary activity often receiving attention and, in many cases, considered as a secondary obligation. This orientation has been one of the paradoxes of our health care system, inpatient versus outpatient care, public hospital versus private facility, and specialist versus primary physician. The hospital based ambulatory care unit has often been forced to function in consort with the emergency service. In many cases the emergency service instead of playing the role of treatment of emergency illnesses and trauma has been required to assume the role of the practicing community physician, particularly at off hours, during the evening, night and week-ends. [34] Thus, if the hospital ambulatory care unit is to become a primary functioning unit within a primary care delivery system, it must be upgraded to equal status with the inpatient clinical departments of the hospital, and must be given equal authority and responsibility for the delivery of health care. Ellwood[66] has recently suggested that hospital based medical groups could function in ambulatory care areas on a contractual basis acting as a nucleus linked in a network with similar ambulatory care facilities throughout the community. For hospitals to become acceptable successful providers of primary ambulatory care, resources and full-time personnel must be assigned to them. [32]

Similar ambulatory primary health care units could then be developed as satellites to the hospital with established referral channels for specialty consultation and inpatient care. Such satellites could assume the form of group practice, health maintenance organizations or medical care foundations.

THE HEALTH MAINTENANCE ORGANIZATION

McLeod and Prussin, in a recent review article concerning the evolution of Health Maintenance Organizations,[66] have called attention to the components that contribute to a successful HMO.

1. *Contractual Responsibility*

   This responsibility is discharged by the provider in a contract with the consumer. Such contractual responsibility could be developed with the central hospital unit or governmental agency to provide health services for a segment of the population or an enrolled group. The contract usually provides for an agreed series of medical and health care services to the enrolled members at an identified cost with provision for total coverage around the clock. Such coverage could be provided in part by the emergency room of the core sponsoring hospital.

2. *Prepaid Component*

   While this is more than simply an indemnity component that provides the mechanism to pay for the care, it must be locally competitive and is delineated and regulated by the contract mechanism, with or without copayments and supplemental payments which might lower the initial premium cost. Such copayments should have no effect on or increase total costs.

3. *Physician Autonomy*

   Within the contract mechanism, the physician group governs its professional activities, directs clinical matters and is responsible for the quality of care in direct reference to the standards established by the core contracting institution or monitoring agent. The primary care physicians would be required to function within the HMO to oversee the full continuum or services and work within the team. The physician group assumes responsibility for assurance of continued service, referrals, feedback and transfer of responsibility as required.

4. *Shared Financial Responsibility*
Incentives to keep patients out of costly inhospital beds and to favor the practice of preventive medicine would be in the interest of efficiency and in keeping with the contract mechanism.

5. *Service Integration*
There should be coordination between the HMO and the contracting hospital so that back-up facilities and inpatient facilities could be provided. There should be a unit medical record system to avoid duplication and assure greater continuity in the care for the individual patient and his family. The distribution of all information about the patient's health and treatment history must be transmitted and available to all units within the system. Individual encounter forms should be considered; however, adequate dissemination of and ready access to patient information will remain a significant problem. A viable information system is critical to any primary care system. The success and acceptance of the family physician has always been his knowledge of his patients, their histories and their problems. As multiple facilities and personnel become involved in the delivery of direct personal health services this knowledge must be available to all involved in the health care process.

6. *Voluntary Enrollment*
While voluntary enrollment in an HMO may not assure complete free choice of physician, it will allow the patient the option of registering at that unit or another unit of the system. To stabilize the system, the enrollment period must be for a prescribed period of time, however re-enrollment and change must remain as patient options at specific times. In a franchise or regionalized system, freedom of choice may be limited and thus a consumer grievance system and/or ombudsman may be necessary to assure patient satisfaction and access to change within the program.

7. *Comprehensive Coverage*
The consumer or his agent (i.e. employer, union, etc.) negotiates a "package" of services at the initial enrollment period. This "package" should be as comprehensive as possible so that out of plan services and thus additional costs to provider and/or consumer are kept to a minimum. Referral from the HMO ambulatory care units to the core hospital or teaching center for ambulatory care services of a more

specialized nature can be arranged as back-up inpatient services from the contracting hospital. The contract could limit abuse of the inpatient services by encouraging through an incentive program use of the ambulatory care units by both the physicians and the consumer. HMOs attempt to answer four requisites for primary health care delivery:

(a) Equalized access
(b) Balance of supply to demand
(c) Organization to improve efficiency by including prevention, health maintenance, cost effectiveness and need incentives.
(d) Utilization of the present system's strength.

Laur[67] believes that HMOs are applicable to many providers and stimulate cost consciousness while submitting to a required spectrum of services for the enrolled population. The question posed by Laur and other authors has been that of the regulatory mechanisms and the need for identifiable physicians. While in some cases regulation is internal through the enrolled population, the providers still seem to have control of the decision-making process. A state health authority and/or contracting mechanism, through the primary provider utilizing standards and requirements established by the contract, could create a better balance and provide a more favorable consumer position. Gee[68] has noted that the HMO mechanism could be extended to home care, thus utilizing a less expensive, easily organized method to deliver care to patients now prevented from obtained home care because of economic barriers and reticence of physicians and hospitals to accept responsibility for them. If such services were coordinated with the ambulatory care unit and the inpatient hospital program, total cost to the community and taxpayers should be reduced. Whatever mechanism is developed for the delivery of primary care, we must incorporate elements of prevention in such a program to benefit from the potential economic savings. Wilson[69] has called attention to the need for further consumer health education to prevent unnecessary use of health services and to encourage patients to assume greater responsibility for some aspects of personal health care. We must develop within a primary health care system incentives for the patient to remain well.

Proponents of the HMO type delivery systems are supporting this concept on the basis of access to high quality, comprehensive medical care at reasonable costs. They note that prevention, early disease detection and treatment are all equally emphasized. The prepayment mechanism, with contract responsibility between plan members and the physician organization, provides for sharing of financial responsibility. Integrated services, voluntary enrollment, and comprehensive coverage with proper use of manpower are other purported advantages in such a fiscal and delivery mechanism.[70]

THE MEDICAL CARE FOUNDATION

The Medical Care Foundation has developed in recent years a limited management system for community health services.[71] A recent HEW publication reviews a number of existing programs.[72] The Medical Care Foundation concept is most often concerned with the quality of care and costs. Such a plan usually is built upon a medical society-sponsored program with the provision of peer review within a continuing pluralistic system. One of the earliest Foundations for Medical Care was developed by the San Joaquin County Medical Society in California in 1954.[73] Incentives for initiating this program were those of adequate reimbursement and the proper review of costs to satisfy the requirements of the third party carriers that there be a review mechanism of possible excessive charges in the delivery of health services.

There is some regulation, through a foundation, by control of fees and by the utilization of consumers, and in some cases intermediaries, on the governing boards. Two types of medical care foundations are currently under development or in existence throughout the United States, usually with county or state medical society sponsorship:

1. *Comprehensive Foundation*

   This type of foundation sponsors a prepaid program with peer review for quality and minimum standards of performance. Standards can be negotiated with carriers and deal with such items as the length of hospital stay, diagnostic procedures, medication utilization, treatment modalities and other criteria of patient care. A committee on fees sets relative values or conversion factors to prevent and/or discourage overutilization and excessive charges. Model treatment profiles are developed and physicians, either in solo or group practice, are encouraged to adjust to the experience of the total group through the mechanism of peer review. Physicians, in most cases, occupy the majority of positions, if not all, on peer review committees and often are paid for such activities. The costs of such peer review programs is between 2.5 and 4 percent and usually these costs are passed directly to intermediaries who save through hospitalization review and reduction in total costs of the delivery of the "package" of services.

2. *Limited Foundation*

   This type of foundation directs itself toward claims review and does not make any attempt to develop or sponsor a health care delivery program. The claims review system is a peer review system and often does not direct itself toward the quality of care but more toward the cost of care and the development of an appeal mechanism.

   At present, there are at least 18 statewide foundations and 43 county foundations, located in 27 states. HR 1, the new federal health law, which became effective July 1, 1973, requires a peer review mechanism directed toward cost savings and the improvement of the quality of care. The foundation system can be adapted easily to this requirement. The San Joaquin Foundation[71] has found that through proper use of physician services, laboratory services, etc., as much as 12 to 15 percent saving on premiums can be realized through reduction in utilization of the more costly health services. Some foundations have used the review mechanism to deny payments for hospitalization when it has not been properly certified or has been unnecessarily lengthy. Many observers, such as Davis,[74] see the foundation as the answer to the threat of control of the practice of medicine by a closed panel system and note that the foundation can act as a buffer between the physicians and the third party payer. Davis also notes that this buffer can be performed by review of:

(a) The need for care
(b) The appropriateness of care
(c) The reasonableness of cost.

Proponents of foundations call attention to the benefits of the free choice of physician, hospital and carrier by the patient, while at the same time leaving the physician free to serve under the delivery mechanism that he chooses. There is no doubt the consumer is provided greater information than in the past concerning his health care; however, foundations may not have an immediate significant impact on the delivery system, particularly the organization of that system for the delivery of primary care. But foundations may provide the evolutionary phase—a stepping stone in the development of a workable health care delivery system. The comprehensive foundation can be adapted to a prepay or risk sharing system with a regional organization that assures access to quality health care for an identifiable geographic population. Although Harrington[75] notes foundations are patient oriented and attempt to control fees while encouraging comprehensive care, the fact that, at least until the present, they have been built on either complete or majority representation by nonprofit medical societies, will limit their effectiveness in the long run. Greater consumer participation is definitely indicated. There is no doubt that certification of hospital admissions, peer review and utilization are productive. These concepts could be reinforced within the contract mechanism utilizing the additional mechanism of the foundation.

FAMILY HEALTH CENTERS

In the past 10 years we have seen the development of Family Health Centers sponsored by the programs of the Office of Economic Opportunity and Comprehensive Health Planning. These units serving as satellite ambulatory care centers, with responsibility and relationships to a core facility, could provide for a geographic organizational network of primary care facilities.

These units could develop into HMOs, prepay capitation programs, or continue on a lump sum contract basis for the delivery of a comprehensive spectrum of services to population groups or geographic areas usually representing predominantly indigent recipients. These Family Health Centers would continue to function as they have under OEO auspices with the removal of some of the costly programs of training or community development that are not directly applicable to the delivery of primary health care services. Family Health Centers should relate to a core hospital for specialty services, consultations, the rarely used or more costly laboratory and radiological procedures and inpatient care. They should develop within their system an outreach program through family health workers, and a home care program staffed by physicians, public health nurses, nurse practitioners and physicians' assistants. The team concept for the delivery of health care would continue, depending on a proper delegation of health care responsibilities to personnel with the levels of training required to maintain quality of care at a reasonable cost. I believe a satellite system of neighborhood health centers with strong relationship to a core hospital facility can provide the proper organizational structure for a primary health care delivery system.

INSTITUTIONAL APPROACHES

Solo Medical Practice—The impact of Medicaid on private care for the poor has not been as successful as initially projected.[77] Recent estimates indicate the use of private physicians has increased from 1 to 10 percent by those with buying power provided through Medicaid. Most patients still use the hospital clinics since many barriers in addition to finances seem to continue to prevent them from obtaining private medical care.

In addition, apparently a number of patients have indicated they prefer the clinics and the quality provided by them to the care they can purchase through private physicians.

While there remain many advocates for the solo practice of medicine,[78-81] due to the personal commitment, involvement and identity of the physician with his patients, there will probably be a gradual diminution in the number of physicians choosing this mode of practice in the future. As medical practice has become more complicated, the solo practitioner's productivity has been reduced and he will either join in a team effort with allied health personnel or in a group effort with other physicians.

Bartholomew[78] feels that the solo practitioner can deliver the most care at the best price, and his inclusion within the primary health care delivery system in the future will depend on his ability to continue to prove that factor. Peterson[36] calls the single personal physician "both outmoded and indispensable."

Group Practice—For many years there has been a tendency to look to group practice as a possible solution to the health care delivery problems of the United States. Many have pointed to the successful results of the Kaiser-Permanente programs[82] and this oft-discussed concept has received much attention. Others have expressed doubts that group practice would solve all of the problems of distribution and availability of care. Weinerman[83] noted that the most successful group practices are those that are large, most efficient, impersonal and fragmented to the perception of the patient. Others have noted the positive factors of improved quality, decreased hospitalization and improved productivity.[35] Some investigators have questioned this experience by claiming selected populations, impersonal care, physician dissatisfaction and elimination of costly services as prohibitive to valid comparison. Many other factors concerning the utilization of group practice make this method an attractive model for a primary health care delivery system. Battisella[84] notes the tremendous fragmentation of health services into many individuals and small groups has caused a lack of coordination. In many cases it may even "have manufactured illness." Rorem in his Review of Private Group Clinics in 1931, recently reprinted,[85] studied 30 private clinics that came into existence between 1918 and 1928. He noted that most of these clinics were developed on the premise of providing continuous, cooperative health care by full time physicians in common facilities. The patients became the responsibility of the group and in most cases income was pooled. The family physician relationship had been encouraged in 50 percent of these clinics with an interest in the provision of primary care. His review seemed to indicate that group practice on a fee for visit basis had not had a significant effect on costs nor had it necessarily increased productivity of the physicians or other team members although for the first time, he did call attention to the more extensive utilization of other health care personnel for the care of patients' problems. Other authors, such as Glasgow[86] point out that many groups have been formed in the past to serve physician needs rather than public or patient needs. This has led to an increase in effectiveness and cost savings for the provider but not necessarily greater productivity or benefits for the consumer. Donabedian[65] has called attention to this same factor particularly in respect to multispecialty or single specialty partnerships. Fifty percent of the groups in the United States today are single specialty with no increase in productivity above solo practice of the individual group members. Madison[58] believes that the insurance industry has been of little assistance in forcing economies in group practice but rather has served as a "passive accommodating force." Mechanisms to encourage use of the health care team approach may alter this drawback particularly in productivity of physicians.

In the late 1920's, Blue Cross accepted the prepayment concept in group practice. In 1932, the Committee on the Cost of Medical Care of the American Medical Association endorsed group practice for the first time. Groups attempt to pool skills for the benefit of patients and the evidence of a sense of responsibility toward these patients seem to be attractive precepts on which the concept was built. In 1900, there were two group practices in the United States and by 1930, 150 had come into existence. The first group prepay practice was developed by Dr. Michael Shadid of the Farmers Union Cooperation Health

Association in Elk City, Oklahoma in 1929.[87] In 1943, 506 groups were identified and in 1969, 6,371 were listed in operation. In recent years the group practice concept has contributed to the development of the HMO and comprehensive Medical Care Foundation concepts. One possible mitigating factor in the even further expansion of group practice and its acceptance by health care professionals has been the lack of role model presented to medical students. Increasing participation by medical students in group practice educational opportunities, will stimulate further interest in the development of this type of health care delivery. One question that constantly arises is the pattern of utilization between patients in prepay group practices and those on a fee-for-service basis. A recent study by Greenlick et al.[88] comparing general registered patients with patients in an OEO Program in the Kaiser Clinics in Portland, Oregon, revealed that the rates and patterns of utilization are essentially the same. Data collected by this group of investigators indicate that the poverty group had an increased rate of visits for emotional problems, particularly among males. There was a greater appointment breakage among the indigent group but there seemed to be a loss of the different patterns of usage when financial and other barriers were removed. The authors seem to feel the difference in behavior related more to access than other factors. Although the group of 1500 patients studied was relatively small, the OEO group did seem to use the services during unusual hours and with more attention toward ambulatory care facilities. Saward,[89] studying the effectiveness of group prepay practice in delivering care to indigent populations noted that a group of Medicare patients enrolled in a group prepay practice buys 1700 days of inpatient care in one year versus 2700 days used by a similar national group buying care as individuals. Others, such as Vayda,[35] have been interested in the functioning of internists in prepay group practice programs since a significant portion of primary care and continual care must be rendered by internists and pediatricians due to the paucity of family physicians. He notes that house calls by physicians functioning in such prepay groups have been gradually replaced by visits to ambulatory care centers with an average of approximately eight patient visits per week and on the weekend. He also called attention to the fact that the fee-for-service system stimulates approximately a 30 percent increase in hospital bed days over prepay programs, although the activities by internists are the same in both prepay and direct pay programs. Vayda[35] felt that most of the resistance exhibited by internists to joining group prepay practice programs is based on ignorance, rather than actual reticence to participate in such programs. Robertson[90] has compared medical care use of a prepay group practice program and a free choice plan, studying public school teachers in a Blue Plan, 1966-67. He noted that the group practice was related by the contract to hospital facilities and the Blue Plan made higher payments to physicians for services rendered to patients in that group. A total of 2700 school teachers made up the study group and the two sections were felt to be comparable by all parameters including education, type of residence, etc. Use of inpatient care was found to be significantly lower under the prepay program. Male utilization had decreased by 19 percent and female utilization by 3 percent. In surgical cases, male utilization was down by 54 percent, female utilization down by 77 percent. Outpatient utilization was much higher in the prepay program for both males and females than those services utilized under the Blue Plan. A great portion of the increase in utilization of outpatient services was apparently due to systematic encounters. Lewis,[91] Gerber[92] and Hill and Veney[93] did not agree with the conclusions reached by Robertson, although Perrott[94] studying federal employees and other similar groups tends to agree with Robertson's conclusions. The decrease in hospital utilization could be related to hospital access for physicians in group prepay practice which had been limited in some cases.

One major problem facing all group prepay practices is the utilization of non-plan services. This apparently differs from 7.2 percent to 10 percent[56, 66, 90] and must be calculated into the overall costs of the program. Development of group prepay practice is oriented toward seven basic concepts:

1. Nonprofit, self sustaining organization.
2. Prepayment.
3. Self-government by medical groups, consumers and third party payers or various combinations.
4. Spectrum of facilities, ambulatory and inpatient with a single medical record in the ideal system.
5. Voluntary enrollment with dual option.
6. Capitation concept.
7. A predetermined, negotiated comprehensive benefit program with assurance of continuity.

Madison[58] stresses the need for primary care to be a central component of such a program. He notes that groups must provide an available physician at all times with a mechanism for night and weekend coverage. The hospital emergency room or ambulatory care department can serve this function. Thus the group located at a hospital, or functioning as a family care team out of a hospital, provides the added parameters of continuity and availability of care. While the fee-for-service multi-specialty group often does not handle general problems, the comprehensive prepay group can call on specialists when necessary through a contractual arrangement thus decreasing the overall cost of a program. Community input into the priorities and services offered by group prepay practice must be increased as in all phases of the primary health care delivery system.

Falk[95] has endorsed the group practice concept as an important component of a national health insurance program. He urges that such groups become part of such a program and be required to include full cost reimbursement for all supportive personnel, continued training, quality control mechanisms and the full spectrum of health services. All prepay group practice programs must be linked to training programs for health professionals and would be probably best served if, at least in some situations, they were attached to medical schools. The schools could assist in recruiting, act as teaching outlets for students, develop measures of quality, eliminate duplication, continue active research and provide role models for defined populations which would tie the schools more directly to their communities and local needs. Greater productivity may not be attained unless the physician is willing to relinquish many of his previously cherished responsibilities to other professionals. Otherwise allied health professionals may merely act as add-ons.[86] Peterson[36] feels that the quality of care and equity of access are best in group prepay practice. However, the group must not be allowed to unilaterally determine the services, population served, location and costs.

Finally Roemer et al.[56] have recently compared the effect of different types of health insurance on various aspects of health care. Out of pocket expense to the family is least in prepay group practice compared to commercial insurance or provider insurance. Benefit effectiveness was greatest in group and provider insurance and least in commercial insurance. Greater satisfaction was found in group insurance with 65 percent of the patients very satisfied and 26.3 percent satisfied. Only 8.6 percent were dissatisfied with services received under group prepaid insurance while both commercial and provider type insurance provided less satisfaction with the availability of health care and more dissatisfaction with its quality. Group prepay insurance seems to represent the highest level of sickness risk, and yet hospital admissions were the lowest as was out-of-plan usage. Prepay group practice, whether proposed under this name or as a Health Maintenance Organization, remains a very attractive concept for the delivery of primary health care on a national basis and further investigation and research into this concept should be encouraged at all levels.

TRANSPORTATIONAL SYSTEM

Any primary health care system will require a functioning transportation system for the transfer of patients between and among the various elements to assure the ready availability of increasing sophistication of health care services as required by the served population. This system should include the emergency care that can be provided by ambulance; the transportation of patients from home to the health centers and/or hospital for diagnostic or therapeutic procedures by mini bus or other vehicle, and the transportation of the health care personnel, family health worker, mental health aide, nurse practitioners, physician assistants and/or physician to the patient in his home.

COMMUNICATION

Communications between all elements of primary health care are divided into two areas: (1) communication of medical, social, environmental, emotional, administrative, and financial information concerning the patient, and (2) emergency communication to assure proper rationalization of the available health services.

A single medical record must be developed which can be transmitted, either through written word or some form of automation, from one unit to another with the transfer of patients. This medical record in the ideal system must be available to all elements of the system at all times to assure the comprehensive nature and continuity of care.

While the availability of the medical record to inpatient services, satellite units, extended care facilities, etc. is most critical for the proper caring of patients and for avoiding duplication or error in the treatment program, transmission of information about patient charges, units of service, types of service, diagnostic procedures, etc. must also be readily available to all elements in the unit.

The development of such communications will provide a major challenge to our technology. But only when we have developed such a communication system will all elements of primary care be properly addressed and will patients be able to enjoy the flexibility of securing proper health services at multiple entry points into the system.

An emergency radio network is currently under development throughout the United States between hospitals, emergency ambulance services, police and fire departments and other agencies responsible for the delivery of emergency care to the population. Further development of this communication system will provide a vitally needed link in the primary health care delivery system.

As noted by McEwin and Lawson,[96] communications must be improved between the hospitals and health care delivery units and between the practicing physician and the hospital based physician. There must be access of the primary care physician to his hospitalized patients even when under specialized care. If such access is not achieved, continuity of care will be sacrificed and the primary physician will become disenchanted.

FINANCIAL MECHANISMS

Many of the systems for the delivery of primary health care currently under examination may not be more economic than the *laissez-faire* system under which we now function. Studies by Sparer and Anderson[97] demonstrate that family health centers deliver care at the same or greater cost than private solo practice. Even clinic care in large urban public hospitals may be more costly. Unfortunately, in many situations we are unsure of true costs due to inconsistent methods of accounting and past practice of loading many inpatient, educational service and other costs on all hospital functions. Only through the development of true, uniform cost centers and accurate identification and allocation of expenses will we accumulate information on the cost of delivering ambulatory primary care.

Recent studies by Roemer *et al.*[56] establish that group prepay practice is most economic with respect to total cost, per capita cost, family unit cost and out-of-pocket expense for the individual and his family or both. An improved system of cost might include the need to distribute medical education costs for students, interns, residents, allied health personnel and inservice activities across a much broader base such as the taxable or insured public, not merely the per diem rate of the sick. No longer should the costs for these educational activities be intermingled with those of the delivery of health care. Although without a doubt there is a relationship between the two, one accrues to the benefit of the total public while the other is related to specific units of health care. The initial costs of new primary health care facilities will probably require front-end funds with subsequent payback through calculated payment schedules at full operational levels. Most previously designed ambulatory primary health care projects have benefited from initial funding from industry, foundations, government or commercial insurance corporations.[46, 82, 85, 89] Operational costs should be borne by full-cost contributions for all elements of care[5] from multiple sources such as premium payments, employee-employer contributions, governmental tax-levy supplements and self-pay assessments. No longer should other activities of the hospital or health care industry be required to subsidize such activities as the hospital based outpatient department[39] or the family health center.

UNIVERSAL HEALTH INSURANCE

Cost is often a barrier to patients seeking health care. For proof we have only to compare the access provided to patients able to afford care in a voluntary hospital to patients who cannot afford it because of medical indigency and who depend on public institutions. The barriers of accessibility, long waiting, lack of appointment systems and the impersonal care often rendered through ambulatory clinics and ward inpatient services have been well recognized for years.[34]

White[6] has stated the need to know more about the effects of payments on patient care utilization patterns before solutions to potential conflicts can be resolved. In addition, it would seem that a national policy concerning support of health care costs must also evolve very soon. Some form of national entitlement must begin to evolve and such a program must be developed in a manner that does not merely stimulate the increased utilization of unnecessary services, but rather provides increased access to health care. In 1972, Falk[5] noted that the financing system must change the organization, not merely be an add-on. He delineated four problems that must be approached by the financing system.

1. National shortages and nondistribution of health care personnel.
2. Increasing costs.
3. Inadequate delivery system for assuring availability.
4. Lack of controls to assure quality and equal distribution.

We must be careful that financial arrangements developed to provide access to primary care do not encourage irrational use by consumers. We have experienced such events in Medicaid and through national health policies developed by other countries, since overutilization can overwhelm the system to the point of stifling its beneficial effects.

Similarly, health insurance with any type of copayment must be carefully developed since requirements for patient first-dollar coverage has been identified as having a depressing effect on utilization and, at the same time, it is extremely hard to administer due to the requirement that the provider collect a fee from the consumer concomitant to rendering health services. The proponents of patient copayments claim this mechanism is a deterrent to overutilization. Universal entitlement is not without risk and certainly presents challenges of a delicate balance in its evolution. A recent report from Canada[98] notes interesting trends in "free" medical care under the Quebec Medicare System. Overutilization seemed to occur for visits without reasonable cause. Hospital and telephone contacts decreased as ambulatory visits increased. Earlier medical care was obtained by a significant number of patients while, most surprisingly, the physician work week decreased about 8½ hours. This finding suggests the need for further evaluation concerning this factor and its relation to overall productivity. It would thus seem that some type of entitlement on a forward projection basis with a prepay component would be the most conducive to proper utilization and access to primary health care services.

McNerney,[99] among others, has noted the need to find a compromise, a middle-of-the-road plan for development of a system of universal entitlement for the United States. Wilbur Cohen,[100] former secretary of the Department of Health, Education and Welfare, noted in a recent speech that successful social reform takes place in an incremental manner. He also noted that all components of the population must be brought together in seeking institutional and political support, and continuity for the success of a National Health Insurance Program. He urged the blend of public and private responsibilities to provide health care with public financing. He felt existing mechanisms provided by the private insurance industry would serve as the intermediaries. The financing mechanism that evolves must have an effect on the delivery system itself rather than merely acting as a payment or review mechanism. To accomplish this, the consumer must have a role in the decision making and priority setting process. The consumer must share this role with the entire spectrum of providers and intermediaries. No longer can we tolerate a system solely oriented toward professionals and providers. We have learned that systems so devised and directed tend to increase costs while failing to improve the delivery system or health potential. A National Health Insurance Program, utilizing both a federal budget encumbrance in the form of general tax levies and contributions from the employer and the employee through payroll deductions, will provide the basis for initial funding as the next step toward national entitlement. Current programs should be gradually reorganized to accommodate this new funding mechanism, and to broaden the delivery of personal health services. The federal government will gradually become the basic funding agent. It will utilize the machinery created by the private insurance industry, with state agencies and regional health planning authorities providing the mechanisms for establishing and maintaining standards and controls. Enactment of national health insurance will not control costs unless such other governmental agencies are utilized. Controls, generally, are not acceptable to the profession, the public or to legislators who have great difficulty making them acceptable to all elements of society. However, only with controls will costs be held in check until competition and a system of incentives becomes effective. The contract mechanism, with proper administration, could provide a possible solution.

FUNCTIONAL MODEL

This paper has attempted to review, in less than complete manner and with limited reference, those elements which may be necessary for consideration in the development of a primary health care delivery system for the United States. An attempt has been made to identify some of the problems, to delineate trends, and to offer solutions. Such a broad based program must receive acceptance from consumers, providers, intermediaries and government, all of whom must be adaptive to a pluralistic system.

It seems appropriate to present a functional plan for development of an organization and administrative structure that could provide primary care for the major portion of our population. Although this plan will make primary health care services accessible and available, it should be understood that any such plan incorporates specialist services, hospital facilities and the entire gamut of health care disciplines currently under consideration. Before such a plan can be presented, two myths must be dispelled.

1. Some political leaders claim that a new primary health care system, utilizing additional allied health professionals and funded by a national mechanism, will be less costly. Such a plan will not provide cheap medical care. Medical care is expensive and the author is unaware of any consistent proof that the cost of medical care for all citizens can be significantly reduced without compromising quality or the spectrum of services provided. Although more care and a greater breadth of services could be provided to more consumers under a more highly organized system, the extension of health care to many unserved and underserved individuals will of itself increase the cost.

2. Some professionals claim that development or greater organization, the team care concept, fixed rates and prepay concepts will diminish quality. No national policy or plan should be developed that will encourage second class medical care. Therefore, the use of additional or new allied health personnel to deliver personal health services should not be at the expense of quality. While priorities may be restructured and decisions concerning access broadened, the nation would gain very little if it sacrificed the high quality of medical practice. Fears of the development of an inferior system must be dispelled by demonstration and fact.

The pluralistic system of health care delivery will be continued in the future and should be maintained to assure freedom of choice not only for the consumer but also for the current and future professional. Only through such choice will we continue to stimulate the most energetic and well motivated members of our society to seek careers in the health professions with the knowledge that they will not be forced into a single career pathway or be limited in their potential for self expression and individual career development. The self-selection process should lead to the choice by consumers of the most responsive mechanism for health care delivery. At the same time incentives and rewards must be developed that will encourage service in areas where access to health care is nonexistent or limited. Each state or region should be required to develop a health authority. This health authority would be responsible for development of a health care delivery plan with rationalization of existing resources and new resources to assure access to all individuals in a designated geographic area and/or population unit.[6, 65] The health authority would have representation from providers, consumers, fiscal intermediaries and governmental agencies, including but not necessarily limited to, state health departments, state comprehensive health planning agencies and educational facilities. The actions of the authority would be implemented by an executive committee, consisting of three to seven persons, representing fiscal, regulatory and educational disciplines responsible for the functional unit.

The executive committee would be charged with enforcing standards, productivity, accountability, performance and evaluation. The authority and its executive committee would be supported by a full time staff responsible for developing, monitoring and negotiating health care contracts between providers, consumers and fiscal intermediaries. The health authority would be responsible for developing a network of primary health care facilities with relationships to consultation services, specialty referral units, extended care facilities and all other elements of a unified health care delivery system. These regional networks would be based on geographic areas and/or population units so that each would be of a manageable size with a unified direction provided by a single central administrative and professional management unit.[46, 47] Management would be directed to properly allocate costs, develop cost effectiveness, allocate the utilization of manpower, implement standards, capitalize on new technology and improve access. The health authority would utilize the contract mechanism to develop a spectrum of services based on a comprehensive health care program developed and confirmed by both the providers and the consumers within each regional unit.

The providers would be oriented toward the hospitals in a region with primary contracts written between the health authority and the hospitals for the provision of health services.

The hospitals would be responsible for subcontracting for the primary ambulatory health care components to various units including hospital outpatient departments, satellite family health centers (either directly sponsored by the hospital or any independent units), Health Maintenance Organizations and Medical Care Foundations. Therefore, groups and individual providers could participate in a relationship with the hospitals through ambulatory care facilities on a subcontract basis and through Foundations as the representative agent. The contract mechanism would be utilized not only to assure the spectrum of services for the consumers, but also to regulate productivity and costs within the system. The providers would share in the risk by agreeing to a total contract cost for an established period of time with an agreed-upon relative value scale for various services in the negotiated package. Back-up services could be similarly subcontracted with extended care facilities, home care agencies, laboratory services and radiological procedures as necessary.

The consumers would be expected to identify the elements in the system in which they will be registered during an identified period of time, and all services supplied to consumers would be provided on a prepay capitation basis. Funding for premiums and out-of-pocket expenses, if any, outside of the negotiated "package," would be the responsibility of the individual consumer. However, the source of payment for both premiums and services might be from general federal subsidies, tax deductions, rebates or personal financial resources. Fee-for-service coverages could be applied within such a system based on negotiated guidelines and with limitations imposed by the total cost of the "package" subject to renegotiation at specific time intervals. The individual and/or family unit would be free to seek health care on such a basis but it would be illegal to combine both methods of payment to a single provider or subcontractor. Within each regional network the health authority would be expected to contract for a transportational system that would include emergency transportation for acute episodes of illness or trauma and continuous transportation system for the transfer of patients between and among the various elements of the program.

Similarly, the health authority would develop standards of communication between the various elements in the system and demand accurate cost center accounting within the communication system which also would deal with patients' medical records and encounter histories.

Each regional unit would be expected to provide for each consumer an identifiable primary health care contact, supplemented and complemented by a team of allied health professionals. Each hospital serving as the primary contractor would be expected to assure continuity of care by providing access to the hospital's facilities to all primary care physicians functioning in the ambulatory care units. Such physicians would have access to their patients as inpatients and would be judged on their ability to render service in the hospital setting.

Specialty care services and/or expensive little utilized services would be centrally located in the hospital facilities or at established units sponsored by the hospitals or subcontractors. Access to such facilities would be available to all consumers and providers based on professional standards rather than owners' rights. Referrals to specialists would be encouraged on the basis of need, with incentive rewards for continued ambulatory care, preventive care and health maintenance. Specialists will be encouraged to act as consultants and prevented from usurping the right of access to individual patients. Hopefully, each regional unit would be identified with a medical school that would assume responsibility for the tertiary care or consultant procedures, recruitment of health manpower, continued health professional education and the development of educational role models for its students. Ambulatory care units would be conducted on an appointment system with full integration of all patients regardless of sources of payment.

Each subcontractor would be required to develop acceptable mechanisms to cover walk-in visits, emergency care and provide full-time coverage including nights and weekends. Such coverage could be supplied by the back-up or primary contractor at the hospital as long as adequate transportational facilities, public or contracted, were available for patients.

Initial subcontracts with new primary care facilities would provide front-end funding to be recouped as maximum operation and total funding are obtained. Educational costs and other nondirect service costs would be removed from the total program costs and supported through other governmental tax based grants and/or contracts.

A grievance or appeal mechanism should be developed within each regional plan so that consumers might voice immediate dissatisfaction concerning services provided and/or quality of care received. The contracts would encourage the use of task oriented personnel and less expensive facilities for the delivery of care. However, at the same time, constant monitoring and a responsive grievance procedure would assure quality of care at appropriate levels for all consumers.

The development of such a primary health care system, building on existing facilities, with the addition of new programs to fill out the network, would capitalize on the positive elements of our existing health care industry, without destroying those programs that have proven to be beneficial and productive in the past. Existing mechanisms of health planning and certificate of need, where available, would be utilized to limit duplication of effort within each network and encourage the referral of patients to higher levels as necessary. In those regions where such procedures are as yet incomplete the health authority would be responsible for refinement and full implementation.

CONCLUSION

Over the next few years we will experience a gradual but persistent evolution in our primary health care delivery system. As we move toward a national program of equal access to health care, based on needs and the right of all society to such access, we will build on various existing elements of the system and through a process of modification, improvement and change the nation will retain a pluralistic industry as a national health policy is formulated. This national health policy will be implemented by the creation of a program of national entitlement based on multiple funding mechanisms administered by the existing insurance industry as fiscal intermediaries. State or regional health authorities, utilizing the contract mechanism, will develop networks of ambulatory primary health care facilities with existing hospitals as focal points of centralized management responsible for subcontracting ambulatory, specialty and extended care facilities, transportational and communications systems. The marked increase in number and categories of health care providers will provide the stimulus to this change which will be implemented at the local level by greater access, a comprehensive negotiated spectrum of services, enforced continuity and a greater emphasis upon prevention, consumer health education and personal health maintenance.

Any new system must take into account the previous roles and future needs of both consumers and providers. The solvency and integrity of the system must be sensitive to the need to build on existing strengths, broaden health coverage to unserved and underserved populations and be aware of the fact that health care is often merely an act of listening followed by a sensitive and knowledgeable response.

REFERENCES

1. Engle, G. L., Must We Precipitate a Crisis in Medical Education to Solve the Crisis in Health Care? *Annals of Internal Medicine,* 76, 487-90, 1972.

2. Annis, J. W., Tomorrow's Health Care Delivery System—What Will It Be Like? Conference on Digestive Disease as a National Problem, Airlie House, Washington, D.C., April 24, 1973.

3. Peterson, O. L., How Effective Will National Health Insurance Be? *Annals of Internal Medicine,* 78, 739-49, 1973.

4. Bergland, R. M., Neurosurgery May Die, *New England Journal of Medicine,* 288, 1043-46, 1973.

5. Falk, I. S., Financing for the Reorganization of Medical Care Services and Their Delivery, in Andreopoulos, S. (Ed.), MEDICAL CURE AND MEDICAL CARE, *Milbank Memorial Fund Quarterly,* 50, 191-221, 1972 (Part 2).

6. White, K., Health Care Arrangements in the United States: AD 1972, in Andreopoulos, S. (Ed.), MEDICAL CURE AND MEDICAL CARE, *Milbank Memorial Fund Quarterly,* 50, 17-40, 1972 (Part 2).

7. Millis, J. S., A Rational Public Policy for Medical Education and its Financing, National Fund for Medical Education, New York, N.Y., 1971.

8. Proger, S., The Evaluation of Different Types of Physicians for Different Types of Health Care, *The Pharos,* April, 1972, pp. 53-66.

9. Kraus, A. S., Botterell, E. H., Einerson, D. W. and Thompson, M. G., Initial Career Plans and Subsequent Family Practice, *Journal of Medical Education,* 46, 827-30, 1971.

10. Gandevia, B. A., History of General Practice in Australia, *Medical Journal of Australia,* 2, 381-85, 1972.

11. Huntley, R. R., Epidemiology of Family Practice, *Journal of the American Medical Association,* 185, 175-78, 1963.

12. Vayda, E. and Kopplin, P., Internists in a Consumer Sponsored Prepaid Group Practice Program, *Canadian Journal of Public Health,* 63, 35-44, 1972.

13. Report on Family Practice, *Journal of the Association for Hospital Medical Education,* 5, 26-28, 1972.

14. Herrmann, T. J., A New Trend in Career Interests Among University of Michigan Medical School Graduates, *Journal of Medical Education,* 48, 451-53, 1973.

15. Sidel, V. W., Feldshers and "Feldsherism," *New England Journal of Medicine,* 278, 934-92, 1968.

16. Rogers, K. D., Mally, M. and Marcus, F. L., A General Medical Practice Using Non-physician Personnel, *Journal of the American Medical Association,* 206, 1753-57, 1968.

17. Rosinski, E. F. and Spencer, F. J., The Training and Duties of the Medical Auxiliary Known as the Assistant Medical Officer, *American Journal of Public Health,* 57, 1663-69, 1967.

18. Sadler, A. M. Jr., Sadler, B. L. and Bliss, A. A., The Physician's Assistant—Today and Tomorrow. Trauma Program of the Department of Surgery, Yale University School of Medicine, Yale University Press, 1972.

19. Stead, E. A., Conserving Costly Talents—Providing Physicians New Assistants, *Journal of the American Medical Association,* 198, 1108-09, 1966.

20. Smith, R. A., Medex—A Demonstration Program in Primary Medical Care, *Northwest Medicine,* 68, 1023-30, 1969.

21. Silver, H. K., Ford. L. C. and Stearly, S. C., Program to Increase Health Care for Children: Pediatric Nurse Practitioners, *Pediatrics,* 39, 756-60, 1967.

22. Somers, A. R. and Somers, H. M., The Organization and Financing of Health Care: Issues and Directions for the Future, *American Journal of Orthopsychiatry,* 42, 119-36, 1972.

23. White, K. L., The Ecology of Medical Care, *New England Journal of Medicine,* 265, 885-92, 1961.

24. Willard, W. R. *et al.,* Meeting the Challenge of Family Practice, Ad Hoc Committee on Education for Family Practice, American Medical Association, Chicago, 1966.

25. Coggeshall, L. T., Planning for Medical Progress Through Education, Report to Executive Council, Association of American Medical Colleges, Evanston, Illinois, 1965.

26. Millis, J. S., The Graduate Education of Physicians, Report of the Citizens Commission on Graduate Medical Education, American Medical Association, Chicago, Illinois, 1966.

27. Peterson, O. L., Andrews, L. P., Spain, R. S. and Greenberg, B. G., An Analytical Study of North Carolina General Practice, *Journal of Medical Education,* 31 Part II, 1-165, 1956.

28. Koos, E. T., THE HEALTH OF REGIONVILLE, New York, Columbia University Press, 1954.

29. Sheps, C. G., Sloss, J. H. and Cahill, E., Medical Care in Aluminum City—I Families and Their "Regular Doctors," *Journal of Chronic Diseases,* 17, 815-26, 1964.

30. Hassinger, E. and McNamara, R. L., Relationships of the Public to Physicians in a Rural Setting, Columbia, Missouri, Missouri Agricultural Experiment Station, Research Bulletin No. 653, 1958.

31. McKeown, T., Organization of Hospitals for Community Health Services and Future Patterns of Medical Care, *The Johns Hopkins Medical Journal,* 124, 271-76, 1969.

32. Connors, E. J., Delivery and Financing of Health Care, *Hospitals,* 46, 71-74, 1972.

33. Weinerman, E. R. and Edwards, H. R., Yale Studies in Ambulatory Medical Care, "Triage" System Shows Promise in Management of Emergency Department Load, *Hospitals,* 38, 55-62, 1964.

34. Weinerman, E. R., Innovation in Ambulatory Services, *Journal of Medical Education,* 41, 712-21, 1966.

35. Vayda, E., The Potential of Prepaid Group Practice in Community Medicine Teaching Programs, *Milbank Memorial Fund Quarterly,* 48, 129-43, 1970.

36. Weinerman, E. R., Research Into the Organization of Medical Practice, *Milbank Memorial Fund Quarterly,* 44, 104-45, 1966, Part 2.

37. Fisher, A. W., Patients' Evaluation of Outpatient Medical Care, *Journal of Medical Education,* 46, 238-44, 1971.

38. Brook, R. H., Berg, M. H. and Schechter, P. A., Effectiveness of Nonemergency Care Via an Emergency Room, *Annals of Internal Medicine,* 78, 333-39, 1973.

39. Deitrick, J. E., Organization of Outpatient Departments, *Journal of Medical Education,* 41, 710-11, 1966.

40. Beloff, J. S., Snoke, P. S. and Weinerman, E. R., Yale Studies in Family Health Care. II Organization of a Comprehensive Family Health Care Program, *Journal of the American Medical Association,* 204, 355-60, 1968.

41. Beloff, J. S. and Weinerman, E. R., Yale Studies in Family Health Care, I Planning and Pilot Test of a New Program, *Journal of the American Medical Association,* 199, 383-89, 1967.

42. Editorial—The Future of Primary Care, *Lancet,* 760, 1325-26, 1970.

43. Primary Medical Care—Report of the Working Party, British Medical Association Planning Unit Report No. 4, 1970.

44. Duncan, B. and Kempe, C. H., Joint Education of Medical Students and Allied Health Personnel, *American Journal of Diseases of Childhood,* 116, 499-504, 1968.

45. Pellegrino, E. D., The Generalist Function in Medicine, *Journal of the American Medical Association,* 198, 127-31, 1966.

46. Weinerman, E. R. and Steiger, W. A., Ambulatory Service in the Teaching Hospital, *Journal of Medical Education,* 39, 1020-29, 1964.

47. Springall, W. H., The Resource Systems Clinical Management Divisions and Group Practice Concept, Temple University Health Sciences Center, Philadelphia, 1971.

48. Durbin, R. and Springall, W. H., ORGANIZATION AND ADMINISTRATION OF HEALTH CARE, C. V. Mosby Company, St. Louis, 1969.

49. The Practice of Personal Medicine, *Editorial, Association of Internal Medicine,* 78, 448-49, 1973.

50. Dean, T. M., Attitude of Medical Students Towards General Practice, *British Journal of Medical Education,* 6, 108-13, 1972.

51. Garrison, G. E., Primary Medical Care—Its Provision Can Be Made Competitively Attractive to Physicians, *Journal of the American Geriatrics Society,* 19, 575-81, 1971.

52. Millar, J. R. M., Primary Medical Care, *British Medical Journal,* 2, 667, 1970.

53. Gilbert, J. R., The Primary Physician: A Unique Role, *Canadian Medical Association Journal,* 106, 1007-10, 1972.

54. Analyn, W. G., Chairman's Address 1985, *Journal of Medical Education,* 46, 917-26, 1971.

55. Crawford, R. L., Reasons Physicians Leave Primary Practice, *Journal of Medical Education,* 46, 263-68, 1971.

56. Roemer, M. I., Hetherington, R. W., Hopkins, C. E., Gerst, A. E. Parsons, E. and Long, D. M., Health Insurance Effects, Bureau of Public Health Economics, Research Series No. 16, 1972; see also Bellin, S. S., Geiger, H. J. and Gibson, C. D., Impact of Ambulatory-Health Care Services on the Demand for Hospital Beds, *New England Journal of Medicine,* 280, 808-12, 1969.

57. Andrews, J. L., Medical Care in Sweden, *Journal of the American Medical Association,* 223, 1369, 1973.

58. Madison, D., The Structure of American Health Care Services, *Public Administration Review,* Sept.-Oct. 1971, pp. 518-25.

59. Somers, A. R., HEALTH CARE IN TRANSITION: DIRECTIONS FOR THE FUTURE, Hospital Research and Education Trust, Chicago, Illinois, 1971.

60. Breslow, L., The Organization of Personal Health Services, First Sun Valley Conference, June, 1971.

61. Cronkhite, L. W. Jr., A Prototype: Massachusetts; Health Inc., *Hospitals,* 45, 71-73, 1971.

62. Heyssel, R. M., Prototypes: Maryland; the Columbia Medical Plan and the East Baltimore Medical Plan, *Hospitals,* 45, 69-71, 1971.

63. Braverman, J., Universities Give New Impetus to Old Concept, *Journal of the American Pharmaceutical Association,* 9, 563-67, 1969.

64. Connor, A. F. Jr., Neighborhood Health Centers and Prepaid Group Practice as a Method of Improving Systems for Delivery of Care in the Urban Core, *Journal of the National Medical Association,* 63, 486-87, 1971.

65. Donabedian, A., Models for Organizing the Delivery of Personal Health Services and Criteria for Evaluating Them, in Andreopoulos, S. (Ed.), MEDICAL CURE AND MEDICAL CARE, *Milbank Memorial Fund Quarterly,* 50, 103-54, 1972.

66. Ellwood, P. M. Jr., Models for Organizing Health Services and Implications of Legislative Proposals, in Andreopoulos, S. (Ed.), MEDICAL CURE AND MEDICAL CARE, *Milbank Memorial Fund Quarterly,* 50, 73-101, 1972; see also McLeod, G. K. and Prussin, J. A., The Continuing Evolution of Health Maintenance Organizations, *New England Journal of Medicine,* 288, 439-43, 1973.

67. Laur, R. J., Four Requisites for Developing HMOs, *Hospital Progress,* 53, 63-65, 1972.

68. Gee, D. A., HMO Breathes Life Into Home Care, *Hospitals,* 46, 39-43, 1972.

69. Wilson, V. E., New Initiatives in Prevention, *Preventive Medicine,* 1, 288-91, 1972.

70. Health Maintenance Organizations, Hearings before the Subcommittee on Public Health and Environment, House of Representatives, Serial No. 92-88, Part 1 and Serial No. 92-89, Part 2, U.S. Government Printing Office, Washington, D.C., 1972.

71. Egdahl, R. H., Foundations for Medical Care, *New England Journal of Medicine,* 288, 491-98, 1973.

72. Experimental Medical Care Review Organization (EMCRO) Programs, DHEW Publication No. (HSM) 73-3017, March, 1973, Washington, D.C.

73. Harrington, D. C., San Joaquin Foundation for Medical Care, *Hospitals,* 46(6), 67-68, 1971.

74. Davis, J. T., The Mississippi Foundation for Medical Care, *Journal, Mississippi-Southern Medical Association,* 13, 332-34, 1972.

75. Harrington, D. C., Foundation for Medical Care, *Journal, Medical Association of Georgia,* 60, 138-40, 1971.

76. Brian, E., Foundation for Medical Care Control of Hospital Utilization: CHAP-A PSRO Prototype, *New England Journal of Medicine,* 288, 878-82, 1973.

77. Olendzki, M. C., Gram, R. P. and Groodrich, C. H., The Impact of Medicaid on Private Care for the Poor, *Medical Care,* 10, 201, 1972.

78. Bartholomew, R. E., The Case for Solo Practice, *Pediatric Clinics of North America,* 16, 939-44, 1969.

79. Burnum, J. F., What One Internist Does in His Practice, *Association of Internal Medicine,* 78, 437-44, 1973.

80. Stone, R. S., The Family Practitioner: A Product of Orthogenesis or Natural Selection, *Journal of Medical Education,* 46, 813-14, 1971.

81. Payne, B. C., The Role of the Primary Physician, *American Journal of Diseases of Childhood,* 116, 468-71, 1968.

82. Somers, A. R., The Kaiser-Permanente Medical Care Program: A Symposium, The Commonwealth Fund, New York, N.Y., 1971.

83. Weinerman, E. R., Problems and Perspectives of Group Practice in Elling, R. H. (Ed.), NATIONAL HEALTH CARE, Aldine Atherton, pp. 212-13, Chicago, 1971.

84. Battisella, R. M., Rationalization of Health Services: Political and Social Assumptions, *International Journal of Health Services*, 2, 331-48, 1972.

85. Rorem, C. R., Private Group Clinics, *Milbank Memorial Fund*, New York, N.Y., 1971.

86. Glasgow, J. M., Prepaid Group Practice as a National Health Policy, *Inquiry*, 9, 3-15, 1972.

87. Shadid, M., The Logic of Cooperative Medicine, *The Social Frontier*, 5, 183-85, 1939.

88. Greenlick, M. R., Freeborn, D. K., Colombo, T. J., Prussin, J. A. and Saward, E. W., Comparing the Use of Medical Care Services by a Medically Indigent and a General Membership Population in a Comprehensive Prepaid Group Practice Program, *Medical Care*, 10, 187-200, 1972.

89. Saward, E. W., The Relevance of Prepaid Group Practice to the Effective Delivery of Health Services, DHEW Community Health Service Publication, 1969.

90. Robertson, R. L., Comparative Medical Care Use Under Prepaid Group Practice and Free Choice Plans: A Case Study, *Inquiry*, 9, 70-76, 1972.

91. Lewis, C. E. and Keairnes, H. W., Controlling Costs of Medical Care by Expanding Insurance Coverage: Study of a Paradox, *New England Journal of Medicine*, 282, 1405-412, 1970.

92. Gerber, A., Letter to the Editor, *American Journal of Public Health*, 61, 901-02, 1971.

93. Hill, D. B. and Veney, J. E., Kansas Blue Cross/Blue Shield Outpatient Benefits Experiment, *Medical Care*, 8, 143-58, 1970.

94. Perrott, G. S., Utilization of Hospital Services under the Federal Employees Health Benefits Program, *American Journal of Public Health*, 56, 57-64, 1966.

95. Falk, I. A., Functional Group Practice in a National Health Program, *Yale Journal of Biology and Medicine*, 44, 153-59, 1971.

96. McEwin, R. and Lawson, W. S., The Communications Gap Between Hospital and Family Doctor, *Medical Journal of Australia*, 1, 1334-39, 1971.

97. Sparer, G. and Anderson, A., Cost of Services at Neighborhood Health Centers, A Comparative Analysis, *New England Journal of Medicine,* 286, 1241-45, 1972.

98. Enterline, P. E., McDonald, J. C., McDonald, A. D., Davignon, L. and Salter, V., Effects of "Free" Medical Care on Medical Practice in Quebec, *New England Journal of Medicine,* 288, 1152-55, 1973.

99. McNerney, W. J., Health Care Financing and Delivery in the Decade Ahead, *Journal of the American Medical Association,* 222, 1150-55, 1972.

100. Cohen, W., Speech—National Health Insurance—A Look Ahead, Princeton University, College of Medicine and Dentistry of New Jersey, Princeton, N.J., March 6, 1973.

DISCUSSION

J. P. MUNSON: John Gardner, former secretary of the Department of Health, Education and Welfare and now director of Common Cause, wrote a book called *Excellence.* His proposition is that we can have both equality and excellence in education. Although this book deals with education in America, with a little revision it could very well be about the health care delivery system.

In their papers Drs. Bergen and Parker are talking about the same basic problem: can we have equal as well as excellent medical care by changing the present system of health care delivery? Their discussion, for me at least, has placed most of the problems of national health in a much clearer perspective.

Rather than discussing Dr. Bergen's presentation in its entirety, I shall discuss his conclusions. Conclusions are always what I read first in any medical article, and if I agree I don't read the rest. If I disagree or have no opinion, I then go back and match my own reasoning against the author's. In Dr. Bergen's case, I both agreed and disagreed so I will give the conclusion as I have rewritten it:

"Over the next few years, we will experience an evolution in our primary health care delivery system. As we are driven toward a national program of equal access, we will use various existing elements of the system to develop an entirely new approach to health care delivery. The approach will be pluralistic, but only on a temporary basis. It will be implemented by universal entitlements based on multiple funding mechanisms. The system may or may not use existing insurance carriers as fiscal intermediaries. Using the contract mechanism, state, regional and local health authorities will develop networks of ambulatory primary health care facilities with existing hospitals as focal points of centralized management. These networks will be responsible for subcontracting ambulatory, specialty, and extended care facilities, transportational and communications systems.

"The marked increase in number and categories of health care providers will act as a stimulus to this change. Under the system there will be greater access to health facilities, a comprehensive negotiated package of services, with enforced continuity and greater emphasis on prevention, consumer health education, and personal health maintenance . . . "

To implement this system, I foresee that some existing barriers or elite controls must give way. Dr. Bergen, in his excellent analysis of the current health delivery systems, skips rather lightly over the issue of controls. These controls would fall into three major areas: 1) competence of the health care delivery personnel; 2) cost of delivery, and 3) consumer involvement in decision making at the national, state, regional and local level (but most of all the last two levels). I call these the three C's of change.

1. *Competency control* of supportive personnel to the local primary physician has not been a serious difficulty. Incompetent nurses, laboratory or X-ray technicians and others are usually weeded out not by their peers, but rather by their masters—the physicians and hospital administrators. The M.D., however, lives in a different world, being judged only by his peers. This is where the present system falls apart, and this is probably my most obvious point of disagreement with Dr. Bergen and the majority of my professional colleagues. Twenty years ago or even more recently, I would have died on the cross of peer review. Today, I say it is a failure, and must be changed to consumer review or at the very least a combination of consumer and professional review.

I have spent the last 16 years sitting on state and local boards of education dealing with public schools, colleges and universities. My change of heart is directly related to my experiences in this capacity. Peer review has failed miserably in our public school teachers. Peer review in our universities and colleges is now on the throes of being dismantled. In both instances, it was because they failed to recognize the rights of the consumer. Twenty-three years as a primary care physician have convinced me that my profession is no more charitable than the profession of education. I don't know how this competency evaluation can be accomplished for we are a tightly knit and wealthy professional union. The times are right for this change, however, for the attitudes of our society as a whole are changing. I believe Howard Simons, managing editor of *The Washington Post,* when he states that the physician with his Cadillac and foreign sports car, his house on the hill as well as a condominium in Florida or some mountain resort, is no longer able to retain his position on the pedestal of public esteem. More than his wealth, however, the physician has destroyed that old Marcus Welby and Rex Morgan image by his or her failure to spend time with the patient during the day, and the use of the answering service in the cold dark fear of night, when his oral counsel is often all that is needed. Aided and abetted by our medical schools, the physician is slowly but surely committing suicide as an independent, uncontrolled member of society. The license and privilege to practice is not a mandate of competency any more than graduating in the top 10 percent of a class is a guaranteed road to success. Competency of a physician can only be honestly judged by the community he serves. Quality control and accountability will only be possible when the competency of the provider is on the line.

2. *Cost analysis* is the second item of control. It must be a vital part of all health care. Which should we choose: $6,000 for six more months of life for a man with renal failure, or the same amount to rehabilitate three children with chronic brain dysfunction? Federal expenditures started the trend with Medicare and Medicaid, but it is a rather sad story that the cost analysis of Medicare shows a stimulus to increase the costs of medical services to all other segments of the population not covered under these programs. Over the period of my time in medical practice, I have seen Medicare, Medicaid, Blue Cross, Blue Shield and NHA triple the cost of primary health care in my community. I request no *executive clemency* for my fees have followed the Blue Shield schedule. Nor have I engaged in a valiant battle to curb the spiraling costs in hospital room rates, lab or x-ray fees. I do not know how to develop a cost-production analysis on such a vague and variable thing as health services, but it must be done before the wrath of the patients being fleeced comes crashing around our heads.

3. *Community control* and consumer involvement must be developed. I have spoken of the 10 physicians and three other members of the healing arts in my community, which by all standards is good. I suspect, however, that at least 25 percent of the population served by this group is in serious need of better health services. It is not geographical access that prevents these people from having adequate health care, but they are too poor to pay, too proud to beg or, in some cases, ignorant of their needs or where to go for their health problems. Only public education can reach this latter group. It can best be accomplished by community participation. I believe we can best gain an equal and excellent health care delivery system by involving the consumer in the decision making process.

■

JOHN L. S. HOLLOMAN, JR.: When I entered the general practice of medicine 25 years ago, I thought that I was prepared to do an excellent job, having been graduated in the upper part of my class from one of the top three medical schools in the country and having had a rotating internship at an extremely busy urban hospital. This training was followed by more than two years of service in the Army of the United States with entry training at the Medical Field Service School. I had a wide variety of responsible assignments while on active duty. Included among them was a period when I was the radiologist at an airbase hospital. I did the cardiology as well, because there were no other specialists available to perform these skilled tasks.

At the start of World War II a physician could still be a good doctor without being a certified specialist. Excellence, then, was not nearly as dependent on certification by a specialty board as it has become today. In fact, many of the specialty and subspecialty boards had not come into existence although the major boards were established. Group practices were considered to be unethical and were fought by organized medicine. The Health Insurance Plan of New York and the Kaiser plans had not come into existence.

With few exceptions, most black physicians and the majority of white physicians were engaged in what was still proudly called the general practice of medicine. A 1942 survey of black physician specialists reported by Dr. W. Montague Cobb (the distinguished professor of anatomy at Howard University and editor of the *Journal of the National Medical Association*) revealed that there were 85 black physicians who held between them the total of 97 specialist ratings scattered among the approximately 4,000 black physicians in the United States. There were approximately 14 partially certified or certified training centers, excluding Howard and Meharry medical colleges, which would accept black physicians for specialty training. Some of these centers accepted black physicians very reluctantly and sporadically. Discrimination against the black patient and physician alike was the shady side of the American Dream. Racial discrimination and segregation were the usual and customary practices of the health professions, as well as the armed forces of a country which was fighting a second World War to make the world safe for democracy or something. Since that time, and on the positive side, *de jure* discrimination against black physicians and patients has almost vanished although *de facto* discrimination remains evident.

With the rapid technological and scientific advances in medicine, it became quite clear the general practice of medicine would become more difficult. Specialization was certainly an easier and ultimately more lucrative way of practicing medicine. The specialist became more disease oriented and had little concern for the total patient except insofar as his own specialized endeavors were concerned. If the patient's illness should cross specialty lines, care was often either incomplete or redundant unless other appropriate specialists could be located and the given care happened to satisfy the doctor's needs. Unless the generalist chose to qualify in some specialty, he was gradually excluded from the hospital staff, and "in-hospital" patient care became the province of the specialist. The new physician was forced to specialize if he wanted to continue his postgraduate growth through the peer associations afforded him in the hospital environment.

When my years of military service ended, I took postgraduate training in internal medicine at a prestigious university medical center. I worked as the admitting physician in another large urban hospital. I subsequently served as chief medical resident at the same hospital where I had done my internship.

With the assistance of several physicians in the community, I opened an office which was complete with a chemical laboratory, a large x-ray unit, an electrocardiograph, and many other pieces of the most modern equipment including physiotherapy units. Although I had surgical experience in the internship as well as in the Army, I elected to omit surgery and obstetrics from my practice.

In the large urban area in which I worked, hospital appointments to the better voluntary hospitals or medical school-affiliated institutions were unknown or very sharply limited to black physicians. In spite of the inability to secure a voluntary hospital appointment, I thought of myself as a nearly complete generalist. I secured an appointment in medicine at the hospital at which I had been an intern and a resident. I worked in that hospital as a consultant in hematology. While in medical school I had been employed in the pathology department as a diener and had thus been afforded some additional pathology experience.

In my generalist office I was assisted by a graduate chemist who was a medical technician with both civilian and military experience. In addition to this very skillful physician expander, I was assisted by a nurse who was also able to do many tasks in the spectrum of primary care. We did home calls for our patients and, when requested, for other physicians. We operated a blood bank, did laboratory work for many physicians, as well as radiology and electrocardiography. I often served the primary care physicians as a diagnostic and therapeutic consultant. My early activities were more or less duplicated by other young physicians in my own and in other areas of the country. However, this pattern of medical practice was doomed because of the rapid growth of specialization.

The exclusion from the "better" hospitals of the generalist or primary care physician became almost complete in many of our larger urban areas. Although it is an infrequently admitted fact, many physicians stayed on in the hospital training situation because they were either incapable of performing in practice, or afraid of the awesome challenge of the general practice of medicine. In some ways, specialization was, in fact, a "cop-out." Some of the depreciation of the general practitioner by specialists was in part due to guilt feelings or to the feelings of inadequacy from which some specialists were suffering.

In the final analysis, however, the most important force on the health care scene, then as now, is money. Physicians are attracted by a number of things which vary from physician to physician. The prospect of making more money more easily is very attractive to most humans, as indeed it is to most physicians.

The organization of primary health care today and in the future will be shaped by money and by the ways in which money becomes available. The increasing demand for primary care will remain a frustrated unfulfilled cry until the factors of money and prestige for the providers of care have been rearranged. The numbers of providers of care must be increased so that the above factors can become more operative. The trend toward specialization has distorted the health care·delivery system at the expense of primary care.

In looking at Dr. Bergen's presentation, I find myself in general agreement with most of what he says, although semantically there are several areas in which I would express my ideas about the organizational structure for primary care differently.

Bergen states:

"There is no doubt that a pluralistic system will and should continue in the United States."

He notes that Somers says:

"This system cannot be sacrificed, nor should it be sacrificed for a totally new care delivery system."

Each of the many components of our health care delivery system has its vested interest and hence, in most instances, is quite anxious for the continuation of its particular component. The improvement of or the restructuring of the health care delivery system is frequently secondary to the protection of vested interests. The lobbying activities of the organized health providers is dramatic proof of this statement. Health legislation has frequently included this concession to the vested interest, the legislation's preamble, "without disturbing the traditional methods of medical practice."

There are many things that are traditionally wrong with our health care delivery system, and they must be disturbed and changed if the problems we face are to be solved. The discrimination between patients on the basis of their pocketbooks or their ability to pay is incompatible with the concept of health as a right. The concept of the private patient and the charity patient must be abolished if high level of quality care is to be obtained for all our residents. Racial, economic and religious prejudice are unhealthy and must be overcome. These undesirable traditions are so firmly rooted or vested in our present health care delivery system that a brand new system designed to meet the present and future needs of patients may be the best answer to the problem.

The dependence of our health delivery system on the importation of large numbers of foreign trained medical graduates, particularly when larger numbers of qualified American trained college students are being annually turned away from our domestic medical schools, is wrong. Many foreign doctors are handicapped by cultural and language barriers. The use of such physicians for primary care in this country is totally inappropriate. It is alien to the concept of a primary physician as we now see it. It poses a barrier for patients already handicapped by poverty, ignorance and ill health.

In the conclusion of Bergen's presentation, he reaffirms his faith in the private health insurance industry and states:

"National health policy will be implemented by the creation of a program of national entitlement based upon multiple funding mechanisms administered by the existing insurance industry as fiscal intermediaries."

I register strong opposition to this statement, believing that the private health insurance industry is indeed a wasteful extravagance which at this point in time can no longer be afforded. For selected groups it has performed some service but it has been deleterious to our health care delivery system and has added greatly to the high cost of medical care. The waste and duplication among the 1800 or more recognized private health insurance carriers is enormous. The illusion of complete coverage can be shattered in many cases by the careful reading of the innumerable pages of fine print which more carefully delimit the exclusions and the contracted "set of comprehensive benefits" that the comprehensive health policy usually promises. In too many cases the illusion of insurance coverage is only shattered when the patient is confronted with the medical bills not paid for by his so-called comprehensive insurance.

The many skills of the numerous individuals employed by health insurance companies can be more advantageously utilized in administrative capacities or a new health care delivery system designed for the benefit of patients rather than for the maintenance of the private health insurance industry.

In a Federal National Health Insurance system, much of the advertising and sales costs would be eliminated. The ideal health care system would be designed to avoid the gaps in coverage that are presently the bane of the patient's existence. Medical need would be the sole criterion for admission to the system. The ability to pay for needed care would cease to be a barrier. The system would be so structured that financial affluence, or lack of it, would no longer distort the system in favor of the rich or poor.

It is my belief that we do have the knowledge of how to develop a health care delivery system. For many reasons we are slowly developing the will to have a health delivery of high quality for all. It is my hope that health professionals can lay aside vested interest and show us the right way.

■

NORA PIORE: It is certainly a great deal easier to design a coherent structure that would assure convenient and equitable access to primary health care, than it is to say how it can be achieved. Dr. Bergen deserves a lot of credit for having tried to deal as much with what is feasible as with what makes the neatest diagram on the drawing board, even though the assignment, "Suggested Organizational Structure," did not require him to resist the temptation to describe Utopia!

He has given these proceedings a particularly welcome frame of reference for this moment in history. His blueprint fits the long range goals—those things we will get back to when the presently dim outlook for federal leadership in tackling refractory and difficult problems improves. But it is also a blueprint which suggests, and can accommodate, some moves that can be made right now, moves that don't have to wait for federal action, and which can be made without foreclosing important long range options.

In that framework I would like to discuss the present and potential role of the nation's 6000 community hospitals in relation to primary care. I will note some of the problems they face in coping with mushrooming demands for services that hospitals were not designed and are not presently equipped to provide. I will also try to advance some proposals about the potential role of hospitals in evolving a rational primary care structure, the part they could play in developing orderly and appropriately staffed primary care centers in the communities they serve, and the leadership they could bring to organizing the regionalized health care networks into which primary care centers must be fitted.

It is clear from Dr. Parker's paper as well as from Dr. Bergen's, that the design of a coherent health care system must take account of two dimensions—a macro system concerned with the medical care of entire populations and, within this, various micro systems, arrangements for the care of individual patients or of sub-sets of the population. These latter cover a very wide range. At one end is the solo practitioner with his informal arrangements for referring patients to a particular set of specialists with whom he is accustomed to work. At the other end of this scale are the organized group practices, whose formalized arrangements are, in effect, a mini-version of the macro system, with opportunity and responsibility to manage a defined sub-set of resources in the combined interests of a defined segment of the population.

The dilemma, of course, is what to do about the people who are stranded in the middle of this spectrum, those who don't have a doctor who "usually" takes care of them, those for whom there is no Kaiser, H.I.P. or G.H.A. group available to join.

A growing number of Americans seem to feel that they want and do not have a regular physician, that they cannot readily get to a doctor when they want to consult one, that they have difficulty putting together advice from a variety of specialists who treat different conditions and different family members. These complaints appear to come from the middle class as well as from the poor, from the young as well as from the aged, in the city as well as in rural areas, though less often in the affluent suburbs than elsewhere. It is hard to get statistical verification of these impressions, but the rising tide of clinic visits in all types of hospitals, and in all parts of the country, and the fact that hospital clinics, once chiefly for the urban poor, are now used by many people for many different reasons, is convincing evidence that these impressions have substance.

Here is some of the evidence:

- The volume of outpatient visits in the United States has risen three-fold since 1953, the first year for which such data are available. This increase has far exceeded the rise in inpatient admissions, and is greater than the growth of the total United States population.
- Last year, hospitals in the United States reported over 200,000,000 visits—almost one for every American. Three quarters of these were to community hospital clinics and emergency rooms. In comparison, between 12 and 15 million visits were made to prepaid community group practices, and one and a half to two million visits were reported by O.E.O. neighborhood health centers.
- The number of outpatient visits has gone up each year since 1953. The fastest rise occurred between 1962 and 1964 when visits climbed 30 percent from 71 to 91 million. After 1964 the volume continued to rise but at a declining rate. However, the rate rose sharply again between 1968 and 1970, when visits went up 17 percent. They have gone up another 14 percent in just this past year.
- While all visits have tripled since 1953, there has been a five-fold

increase in visits to emergency rooms. These now account for just under one-third of all hospital ambulatory visits, compared to 20 percent in the earlier year. Despite this spectacular rise in emergency room use, traditional outpatient clinics continue to be the principal providers of hospital ambulatory care in the nation, accounting for two-thirds of all visits to all community hospitals.

- Rising clinic use has occurred in hospitals of all sizes and in all parts of the country. One half of all clinic visits today are to hospitals with 300 beds or less. But a quarter of all visits are to the clinics of the 200 largest, mostly urban, hospitals, those with 500 beds or more. Two thirds of all visits are to the nation's 3,430 voluntary hospitals, 30 percent to the 1,621 local public hospitals, and about 4 percent to the 769 proprietary hospitals. While clinic use continues to go up in both voluntary and municipal hospitals, voluntaries today provide a larger share of all visits, 69 percent compared with 61 percent in 1954.

- In 1969 hospitals in the 50 largest United States cities accounted for 46 million visits—40 percent of the United States total. Forty million Americans live in these cities—20 percent of the population. At the same time, 20 percent of all visits are made to hospitals in nonmetropolitan areas, where one third of the United States population is located and where, on average, there are 68 M.D.s per 100,000 population compared with the metropolitan average of 143 per 100,000 population.

  While little systematic information is available on the true costs of hospital outpatient services, and especially on appropriate allocations of hospital overhead to the cost of these services, it is clear that the costs have risen steeply. House staff, once paid subsistence allowances, now receive quite respectable salaries. Attendants and unskilled hospital employees whose below-minimum wages were once heavily subsidized by supplementary welfare payments, are now largely covered by minimum wage legislation and collectively bargained contracts. At the same time, outpatient service revenue has also increased.

- Prior to 1966, outpatient departments were chiefly a charity service for indigent patients, and as late as 1966, clinic charges generally ranged between 50 cents and $5. By 1968, revenue from services to outpatients accounted for more than seven percent of all voluntary hospital patient revenue. It continued to rise, per visit and as a percent of total hospital income, increasing 70 percent in 1968-1970, compared with a 50 percent rise in revenue from services to inpatients. Average revenue per visit in the United States as a whole rose from $10 to $14, a 42 percent increase in that two-year period, and the outpatient component of total voluntary hospital revenue reached eight percent by 1970. It is higher today.

- Only 15 percent of all community hospitals are affiliated with medical schools or accredited as teaching hospitals. These are estimated to account for about 30 percent of all hospital clinic visits. The proportion of hospitals with affiliations rises with size of hospital, from four percent of those with less than 100 beds to more than half of the over-500 bed hospitals. Thus, 85 percent of all outpatient visits are outside the orbit of academic medicine.

What do these numbers mean? What do they all add up to? I think they mean that the greatest hope for improvement in the provision of ambulatory care for millions of Americans must lie in the reform and reorganization of hospital based clinic services, within or outside the hospital premises, but relying and capitalizing on the unique ability of the hospital as the one institution in our society in a position to mobilize resources and attract, organize and deploy the doctors, nurses and allied workers who have the training and the skills to maintain health and treat illness.

The shortcomings of hospital clinics, from the viewpoint of the patients who seek care in these clinics as well as from that of the physicians, nurses and aides who provide it, are too well known to require repetition here. Many students of health affairs are convinced that no way can be found to alter and improve hospital outpatient departments, so that they can become satisfactory primary care centers. The dilemma is that none of the alternatives that have been proposed and tried out have taken hold and succeeded in filling the gaps in service, except in a limited number of experimental situations.

Increased individual medical purchasing power in the hands of the aged and of low income families, through Medicare and Medicaid, have attracted only a few practitioners to undertake to care for the underserved populations. I think it quite unlikely that new types of health practitioners, whether nurse-pediatricians, or physicians who belong to the new Academy of Family Practice, whether they are recruited from the minorities or the poor or the middle class, and whatever their dedication to medicine or to a great society, will have a sustained interest in such a practice, except in a setting that offers an attractive professional environment and opportunity for an acceptable personal life style.

Hospitals can make such a setting possible.

Beyond the Medicare and Medicaid effort to enable people to get to doctors by giving them better medical purchasing power, the most dramatic approach to creating an alternative to the hospital clinic has been the Neighborhood Health Center movement. A major goal of the War on Poverty was to establish 800 such centers to provide care for 20 million urban poor estimated to be without adequate or satisfactory health services. Today, O.E.O. centers offer service to about half a million registered persons and provide something like a million and a half visits a year. Their continued existence depends on the fragile ability of the Congress to renew funds for their operation each year.

Aside from this political hazard, there is also a danger that the quality of free standing clinics will deteriorate once the initial enthusiasm wanes.

Once before in American public health history a flourishing independent dispensary and clinic movement arose as part of the pre-World War I reform wave, to serve the urban underprivileged. By the mid-twenties, a then young, crusading social worker named Michael Davis made an investigation of these free standing clinics for New York City. He found, in a now famous report, that the initial advantages gained by separating out ambulatory clinics from their subordinate position in the hospital hierarchy were before long dissipated as they failed to attract qualified staff without the incentive of hospital affiliations. The issue is not the quality of a health center at the time when it is first initiated, with the glow of innovation, under the inspiring leadership of a Jack Geiger or a Harold Weiss or a Sam Wolf, at a time when the "best and the brightest" of an academic-medicine generation were drawn to the social action scene of the 1960's.

Rather the question is what a network of free standing clinics will be like five or maybe only three years later, when the trumpets are sounding for some entirely different parade, when the primary care clinics may have become merely isolated efforts to cope with the most discouraging, the least rewarding aspects, of the ills that beset mankind.

This does not mean that we should not be setting up neighborhood primary care centers. But it does mean that they must be spliced into a total health care system, in such a way that the tasks of this part of the system cannot be hidden from view. Thus, I am arguing not against the neighborhood health center model, but rather for its inclusion in a structure that can sustain the quality of primary care services long after the experimental period and the halo effect have worn off.

Again, it seems to me that the community hospital offers the possibility of such a structure, supervising and rotating staff to satellite clinics if need be, furnishing membership in a professional community to personnel, back-up and referral resources to patients.

We turn next to the prepaid group practice plans as an alternative for providing care for the people who make up the hospital outpatient load. The history of these plans goes back to the mid-thirties. They experienced their most rapid growth during the Second World War and in the immediate postwar years. There are 24 or 25 group practice plans in the United States today, with probably about 5,000,000 subscribers. It seemed for a while as though the Health Maintenance Organization concept would be the vehicle for spurring a broad and rapid expansion of prepaid group practice alternatives along the lines of Kaiser. But it now appears that HMO support likely to emerge from legislation will be small in volume and, more important, possibly coopted by the proprietary sector, effectively creaming the market and further diverting physicians and resources from those areas where they are now in shortest supply.

If any of these proposals, neighborhood health centers or Health Maintenance Organizations, are to materialize as more than a handful of experiments, a way must be found to build them into a health care structure that can reach all Americans in all parts of the nation. The logical structure, it seems to me, is the existing institutional network of community hospitals. Their clinics already serve large populations, and have the capability to mobilize health manpower and health resources. If the climate was favorable, the time ripe, federal legislation could accomplish this by a very simple formula: any community hospital claiming reimbursement for a substantial volume of outpatient services could—in order to qualify as a provider under Medicare, Medicaid or any proposed national health insurance scheme—be required and assisted to develop and offer a prepaid comprehensive health care option to persons in the catchment area who elect to enroll in such a program. Nothing like this is about to happen right now.

Meanwhile, however, community hospitals are being pushed to a growing concern with ambulatory care and concomitant problems by internal dynamics, by external pressures and by the fiscal and staffing crises which have occurred as consumers have voted with the feet to elect hospitals for this role, simply by turning to hospital clinics in mounting numbers when they cannot find a doctor, or because they have greater confidence in the capability of the hospital to deal with their problems.

I was asked by the Forum to do this reactor paper from my "special perspective." I presume it was meant the perspective of the Columbia Center for Community Health Systems. Establishment of that Center a year ago was Columbia's response to the pressures experienced by all medical schools during the last decade, to reconcile the mission of training scientifically and clinically excellent physicians, with growing demands that they become involved in primary health care of communities immediately surrounding the schools and, simultaneously, abandon their traditional aloofness from public policy controversies regarding the financing and organization of medical care in our nation.

The mission of our Center is to provide a conceptual framework and technical assistance to the efforts of six large hospitals affiliated with the medical school—five urban, one rural—to design and bring about what is hoped will be far-reaching changes in their institutions. The purpose is to bring hospital based services into better alignment with the changing needs of the ever increasing thousands of patients who seek care, especially, though not solely, those who come through the clinic and emergency room doors in search of primary care.

The hospitals are contemplating internal changes in the staffing, financing and general organization of services. Our studies show that our hospitals do not have one single outpatient population, but instead several different constituencies. For many, the hospital is a chief, perhaps the sole, source of care for commonly occurring ailments as well as emergencies. For these families we hope to develop team practice modules, combining the advantages of a private office practice, including opportunity for telephone consultation, with the additional benefits of the hospital resources as needed, adding nurse practitioners to the personnel.

Other clinic uses come because of the special competence of the hospitals to deal with a particular illness—patients with asthma, cerebral palsy, sickle cell disease, who are followed in specialty clinics. Still other patients are referred for a consultation by well baby stations and schools, and by practitioners in the neighborhood who want another opinion or lack the resources to deal with complicated problems.

Still others who cross the hospital threshold are found to get their ordinary care somewhere else, from a practicing physician or a neighborhood center or group clinic, but who bypass these providers when they think they have a serious problem. Increasingly, people have come to have high regard for the scientific competence of hospital staffs. "If you are really sick, you may have to wait for hours but once you get to see the doctor he'll know what to do," is what we hear on the clinic benches, along with the restlessness and irritation at the inconvenience.

No one system of patient triage or organization can appropriately handle all these different constituencies. A way must be developed to sort them as they cross the threshold, and to organize appropriate subsystems for each. It is not so hard to design such subsystems for an enrolled population, as they have been designed already for Kaiser, separating the worried well from the really sick, etc. But how to design efficient arrangements for a self-selected population in an "open" system is quite a different problem. Nevertheless, unless and until it is possible to district hospitals and restrict clinic use to defined enrolled populations, the challenge is exactly that of incorporating the planning features of a "closed" system into the present wide open one.

The hospitals and the Center at Columbia are also concerned with the macro part, the appropriate responsibility of the hospital for the total health needs of the population in its catchment area—those who don't come but perhaps should, as well as those who cross the hospital threshold.

The hospital is seen as having both the responsibility and the opportunity for developing a network linking all providers serving the same population, and of designing an appropriate and effective role for the hospital within this network. In New York City the elements in this potential network include Health Department well-baby stations and school health services, TB, VD, tropical disease and chronic disease control and detection centers, neighborhood health centers and other free standing clinics, as well as solo and group practitioners for whom the hospital is specialty and referral back-up resource.

Of course institutions do not change easily, not even institutions that want to change. Hospitals today face a host of problems in trying to adapt to current circumstances. The typical hospital is inappropriately structured in almost every respect for the volume of primary care it is today called upon to provide.

It is physically designed for inpatient care, with space for mushrooming outpatient services too often crammed into a corridor, inadequate for efficient rendering of service, depressing for the sick seeking treatment, discouraging for those, like the pregnant mother, who should be seeking preventive care.

The fiscal structure of the hospital was designed for inpatient services. Its entire costing and pricing system and income maximizing efforts are geared to caring for bed patients. Only with the advent of Medicare and Medicaid did hospitals begin to consider the possibility of recovering, in separate revenues, the cost of ambulatory services. When these funds became available, hospitals for the most part simply adopted cost justification procedures that would maximize total hospital revenue rather than contribute to an understanding of the most efficient and cost effective, or least costly, system for providing ambulatory care.

The record and billing systems of hospitals are also designed for capturing information at a pace geared to the patient who will be available in bed for several days, and are adequate for feeding information back to a physician on rounds with time to stop at the nursing station to look at the chart. Such a pace is entirely inadequate for either the capture or the retrieval of information regarding the ambulatory care patient whose time in and out is, or at least should be, an episode of minutes rather than days.

Last but not least a major problem is appropriate staffing. To begin with, reliance on house staff interested in differential diagnoses and esoteric diseases to provide routine primary care is a constant source of staff and patient discontent. Next, innovative use of nurse-practitioners and other new health workers has been inhibited by hospital custom which is slow to change. Finally, the system of granting inpatient admitting privileges to private practitioners, in exchange for free care rendered on wards and in clinics, will become more and more obsolete as public and private insurance coverage expands. When income from patient services covers the cost of service, a charity way of paying for service will no longer be appropriate. Already hospitals are moving toward salaried and per session paid attendings. These are fairly specific problem areas, and many hospitals are beginning to recognize and cope with them. But much broader and more basic questions are beginning to crystallize and draw public attention. These are issues centering around the regulation of hospitals and their governance in our pluralist society.

Hospitals in the United States have a strange duality of institutional personality. On the one hand, they represent public capital. Whether through hospital fund drives, real estate tax exemptions or construction grants from tax funds, they have been largely built with public money. Their operating expenses are now covered, in very large part, by third party payments from public sources. The philanthropic contributions. that once played a major role in hospital support now account for only a fraction, though an important fraction, of hospital income. Yet much of the greatness of many institutions is a heritage from the initiative, dedication and leadership of private persons—trustees, medical boards, volunteers—and these groups are concerned to protect the fiscal and scientific integrity of the institutions they helped to build. At the very same time, new non-governmental forces are emerging to represent the people who depend on the hospital for primary care, to speak in the name of these consumers. They also regard the institution as "belonging" to them, though stable and democratic community-organization structures and decentralized community planning agencies are in the early stages of development. Can the strengths deriving from the older philanthropic tradition be married with the new vitality of neighborhood social structures? Can both be conserved while hospital resources are more systematically woven into a coherent health care structure, governed in the general public interest, which must sometimes override the preferences of individual hospitals and resolve conflicts between localities? These are hard questions.

What the country seems to need now is a contemporary Flexner Report, one that would focus on the hospitals' role in contributing to and participating in a rational health care delivery system. The Flexner Report was the outcome of a chain of events, the culmination rather than the beginning, of a movement for the reform of medical education, as Dr. William Kissick has pointed out in his history of that era. That movement began with the founding of the American Medical Association as an organization committed to improving the quality of medical practice through legislative imposition of licensure requirements. Soon, thereafter, President Elliot of Harvard was urging that education of physicians was too important to be tolerated as a proprietary venture—a position for which he was publicly censured by the local medical society. Despite these rumblings of opposition, the movement continued to gain momentum. The Association of American Medical Colleges was established and undertook to set standards for accreditation together with the AMA Council on Medical Education. They sought the help of the Carnegie Institution for the Advancement of Teaching, and Dr. Abraham Flexner was asked to undertake the now famous study of the education of physicians.

Dr. Flexner visited 155 medical schools in the United States and Canada. At Johns Hopkins he found an educational style which combined the German basic sciences approach with the clinical approach of the London teaching hospitals. To this, Flexner added the American Land-Grant College concept, the third element in the package which became the Flexner model.

That the *New York Times* ran a front page story on the Flexner Report on the day it was released is a measure of the public awareness of and interest in the problem at the time, and of the country's readiness to receive and act on those recommendations.

When the report was completed, Flexner moved from Carnegie to the Rockefeller Foundation and, with Rockefeller money, travelled through the country from one medical school to another, using these funds as an incentive to get the medical schools to establish full time chairs of clinical medicine with an endowment sufficient to provide the salary for the incumbent on a full-time basis.

Thus, the scientific model of medical education, which revolutionized medicine in our times, was almost a century in the design and implementation.

In many respects we are already part way into another such century of change, this time in the organization of medical service. Many hospitals in the academic orbit have been engaged in the search for new medical service styles for some time—Yale, Western Reserve, Johns Hopkins, Rochester, Harvard. Perhaps of greater significance, scores of hospitals among the 85 percent that have no medical school connection or teaching affiliation, are also seeking ways to change clinic and emergency room services, and their community roles. They are applying to the foundations for study grants and, in the last few years more than half the applications for Hill-Burton money have been from hospitals wanting to renovate or construct clinic space, and to make rental space available for hospital staff wishing to set up group practices.

In sum, then, a great deal of change is occurring in the organization and delivery of American health services. The issues, for the moment, revolve around primary care. Because so much of the void in primary care is being filled, by default, by the hospitals, and also because the hospitals are the chief social institution in a position to mobilize and deploy health resources and manpower, they are a logical focus for the design and achievement of a coherent health care structure. Such a structure might encompass micro systems to deliver service to individual patients, and able to negotiate networks leading toward a systematic macro structure concerned with health care for entire populations. Thus, the system would move toward the goal of Regional Health Care Authorities, which has been a consistent goal of American health legislation since inclusion of the State Plan Titles in the Hill-Burton legislation of the 1940's.

I think that Dr. Bergen would agree, and I certainly would argue, that ultimately no Regional Health Authority without sufficient statutory mandate to resolve conflicting interests among hospitals, professional organizations, employee and consumer groups, will be really able to manage health affairs and achieve some rational order, while allowing scope for pluralism and for the dynamics of changing technology, advancing medical knowledge and changing social preferences.

Meanwhile, while the federal government marks time, and spontaneous change slowly occurs, the great foundations, searching for the cutting edge that could make a difference, might well find it in a Flexner type report. Such an undertaking would explore the models, in both the macro and the micro dimensions, that have been talked about at these proceedings, and provide technical assistance and leadership as well as money to accelerate incremental changes. At the same time the report would accumulate the wisdom and the material that must be ready for writing the "whereas" clauses and the "be it enacted" clauses, when the times are ripe for the next cycle of federal initiatives.

III THE ECONOMICS OF PRIMARY CARE

CHAPTER 4 • KAREN DAVIS

Financing Medical Care:
Implications for Access to Primary Care

The 1960s brought a significant expansion in federal financing of medical care. The Medicare and Medicaid programs initiated in 1966 are expected to pay $17 billion in fiscal year 1974 for individual medical care services received by the poor and the elderly. These programs have two major objectives: (1) assuring that those covered by the programs receive adequate medical care, and (2) eliminating the financial burden of medical care expenses for covered persons. While Medicare and Medicaid have undoubtedly not been completely successful in meeting these goals, it is clear that the poor have made gains in the use of medical care services relative to other groups and that many elderly would have been encumbered by exorbitant medical bills without the Medicare program.

Rising medical costs and inadequate private health insurance coverage for persons not covered by Medicare and Medicaid have led to pressures for new initiatives in the financing of medical care services. Plans to expand the federal role in financing medical care services are generally concerned with one or more of three objectives: (1) ensuring that everyone has financial access to essential medical care regardless of income, location, or type of family; (2) protecting everyone from medical expenses that are high relative to income; and (3) reducing costs and encouraging efficiency in the delivery of medical care. Since failure to obtain adequate medical care is often closely linked to financial status, several proposals place a special emphasis on assuring access for the poor and near-poor. Others focus on the financial burden of medical care which can affect even middle and upper income families. Some plans attempt to meet both objectives of assuring financial access for the poor and preventing financial burden with a single program. Other financing proposals would attempt to restructure the health delivery system through complete federal financing of virtually all medical services for all citizens.

In spite of considerable debate on various alternatives in the last few years,

157

little consensus has been reached on even such fundamental issues as the emphasis to be placed on various objectives. The means by which these objectives can best be achieved continues to be a major source of controversy. Rather than attempting to encompass the entire range of debate, this paper will focus on the problem of access to primary medical care. Two major questions will be investigated: (1) how successful have existing financing programs been in ensuring adequate and equitable access to primary care for covered persons? and (2) how should new financing programs be designed to help overcome remaining barriers to primary care access?

ACCESS TO PRIMARY CARE

Before turning to an examination of existing financing programs, it is useful to discuss exactly what is meant by access to medical care, what are the major barriers to access to medical care, and what social goal is implied by the phrase, "assure that everyone has access to medical care." What special issues are raised by the question of access to primary care—as opposed to medical care generally?

What Does Access Mean?

Access to medical care has been used in numerous, somewhat confusing ways. For some, access is strictly a financial phenomenon—and means simply assuring that medical care is not too expensive for individuals to obtain. Implicit in this is that many persons—particularly those with low incomes—will not purchase an "adequate" or "acceptable" level of medical care without some financial assistance.

Others distinguish between financial and physical access, and define physical access in terms of the availability of medical resources—for example, how many, if any, physicians practice in a given area. This definition of physical access is fraught with many difficulties. First, how is the geographical region to be defined? Second, once an area is decided upon, should all medical resources be counted equally—or should they be weighted by the distance or time involved in reaching them? For example, if a county is the appropriate geographical area, are all physicians within the county considered to be equally available? If a city is the area considered, are all physicians, both those on urban transit lines and those not in easy reach by urban transit, equally available? Third, should all medical resources be counted or just those within the financial range of residents? Does an abundance of physicians in Central Park West mean that residents in that area have easy physical access to medical care?

Closer examination of the concept reveals that it is really meaningless to talk of physical access solely in terms of numbers of available medical resources. After all, medical care services are, in fact, available to most persons at a cost (including both the price of medical care and the time and transportation costs of attaining the care). If necessary, one could travel 5, 10, or even 100 miles for care—and if medical services are available more cheaply at more distant locations, some persons may be quite willing to incur the travel costs involved in seeking out care over a wider area.

Physical access, therefore, should be conceptually measured not in terms of the numbers of medical personnel or facilities available, in an arbitrarily determined geographical area, but in terms of the monetary and non-monetary costs of obtaining care—the transportation, time, and search costs incurred. If the care required is emergency care, the time cost may be quite high in terms of pain suffered waiting for treatment or higher probability of death or disability.

Viewing the problem in this way should lead to better national policies to improve physical access. For example, if the costs of increasing the supply of physicians in rural areas are higher than the costs of transporting patients to physicians in urban areas, the latter action may be preferable. Furthermore, insuring physical access in monetary terms should raise the possibility of tradeoffs between improved financial access (reducing the price of medical care to the patient) and improved physical access (reducing time, travel, and search costs).

In addition to financial and physical access, attitudes of patients and providers may also pose barriers to access. If individuals fail to seek treatment out of fear or ignorance about the efficacy of care, one may argue that the care is not truly accessible to them. If hospitals or physicians refuse to treat certain types of patients or treat them in an undignified, inhumane way in order to discourage such patients from seeking further care, health care may be considered equally inaccessible. Again attitudes of providers and patients as a barrier to care bear some relationship to the concept of financial access since there may exist *some* price (although perhaps quite high) which will induce providers to render care in the manner accorded more favored patients. Presumably, there is also some bribe price at which the most fearful person could be induced to seek care—so that even fear or ignorance could be overcome with some monetary persuasion (although there may be lower cost methods of achieving the same result—such as through educational programs).

Since physical and attitudinal barriers to access may be reduced by financial interventions, a monetary concept of access (broadly defined) may be used to encompass the whole spectrum of access dimensions. Moreover, the design of a financing program should consider ways in which non-financial barriers to access may be influenced by a financing program. Policies to increase utilization of medical services by directly affecting physical and attitudinal barriers to access should be weighed against policies which increase utilization by paying for medical services.

What is the Social Goal with Regard to Access?

Two quite different meanings are frequently attached to the social goal of ensuring access to medical care. The first is that for a given health status all persons should receive some acceptable level of medical care. The second emphasizes equal access: for a given health status all persons should have the same level of medical care.[1] In many ways, this discussion is analogous to the debate regarding poverty and the distribution of income. Should public policy simply be directed toward assuring that everyone has some adequate level of income—or is there also a direct concern with the *inequality* of after-tax income?

The principal thrust in the income maintenance area has been in defining an adequate level of income. Two approaches have been taken. One approach has been to cost out a minimum, essential basket of goods and services which a family requires, and to set the minimum income at this level. Another approach recognizes that an acceptable level of income is not a fixed, absolute amount (even in real terms), but varies with the level of income enjoyed by society as a whole. Suggestions have been made for varying the "acceptable" level of income with the median income of all persons—for example, setting the poverty income level at half the median income for all families.

Although the principal concern in the poverty area has been with bringing poor persons up to some acceptable income level, there is also a concern with the inequality of income *per se*. Although few persons in the U.S. advocate equalizing after-tax incomes, there is a concern that the distribution of income should at least not become more unequal over time, and some reduction in extreme inequality of income is generally considered desirable.

While equalizing use of medical services has considerably wider appeal than equalizing incomes, it seems likely that the major interest in the U.S. will be with bringing individuals with inadequate medical care utilization up to some acceptable level rather than with minimizing unequal utilization of all persons, given health status. Should differences between high income and low income persons become extreme, however, policies to divert medical care services away from higher income persons might gain in appeal.

Just as in the case of defining poverty income, determination of an acceptable level of medical care is extremely difficult. An acceptable level, of course, could be defined to be equal to that of the maximum current use of medical care. This frequently takes the form of arguments that physician visits per capita, say, should be the same in every state as they are in the state with the highest level of utilization. While this is unlikely to be the basis of social policy for the near future, just as in the case of income maintenance the median level of medical care received by all persons may serve as an indication of the appropriate and feasible level of care of which lower income persons may be assured. For example, for a given health status, physician visits per capita should not be more than 10 percent below the median level. This may be true of quality as well as quantity of care—with the acceptable level of quality bearing some relationship to that enjoyed by higher income persons.

Another definition of acceptable level is in terms of medical necessity—additional medical care is desirable so long as it contributes in any positive way to the state of health. If the state of health is defined quite narrowly, the acceptable level may only be in terms of the "life prolongation" effects of medical care. For example, the Administration recently justified the proposed elimination of adult dental benefits under the Medicaid program on the grounds that absence of dental care does not lead to death.[2] Even if state of health is defined more broadly, the acceptable level of care may not involve the luxuries (such as private hospital rooms or cosmetic surgery) which the rich may demand.

Another viewpoint is that the acceptable level should be defined in terms of the level of use at which the social benefits derived from medical care equal the social costs of providing that care. Social benefits may arise from tangible benefits (such as the reduction in contagious diseases made possible by immunization), economic benefits to society (a healthier work force leads to a more productive economy), or altruistic benefits (all persons feel better knowing that everyone has adequate medical care).[3] This viewpoint emphasizes that provision of medical care requires resources—physicians, nurses, facilities—and these resources could be used in alternative ways (for example, as researchers, educators, schools). Devoting more resources to medical care means that society has fewer resources available for other socially desirable goods and services (some of which may even be more useful in improving health status, such as pollution control, education, etc.).

Therefore, it is not desirable that medical care utilization be pursued to the point of any positive benefit, but only to that point which is justified in terms of the opportunity cost of the resources required to provide medical care services. While this approach is undoubtedly the least operational, it is the underlying concept which will be used in the final section of this paper when we derive an appropriate design of financing programs. Much of the analysis holds, however, for an acceptable level of care defined in other ways.

Access to Primary Care

Unlike specialized medical care, the benefits of primary care tend either to be less crucial to health status, narrowly defined, or to have an impact on health status only over a longer period of time. A portion of primary care serves to relieve discomfort or reassure patients concerning the nonserious nature of illness—rather than immediately abating life-threatening conditions. Preventive care or early treatment of illness may have a more significant impact on prolongation of life or reduction in disability but these benefits may be apparent only over a longer period of time.

As a consequence of the nature of benefits of primary care, barriers to access may be more consequential for primary care than specialized care. If an individual requires a surgical operation to relieve intense pain or prevent death, normal barriers to access are likely to be overcome. That is, in such a situation an individual will ivnest more time and money in obtaining the necessary care even if it requires dipping into lifetime savings, incurring significant debt, or traveling long distances.

In the case of primary care, however, monetary and nonmonetary costs of care may cause the individual to endure minor discomfort, ignore warning symptoms, delay treatment, or do without preventive care. Failure to recognize the potential benefits of preventive care or early treatment may lead to higher future costs.

It might be expected, therefore, that financing programs would induce a greater change in use of primary care services than in specialized care. Unfortunately, data on physician care available from existing financing programs do not typically differentiate between primary and specialized care. The following section, however, examines available evidence on use of physicians' services under existing financing programs.

IMPACT OF CURRENT FINANCING PROGRAMS ON ACCESS TO PHYSICIAN CARE

The Medicare and Medicaid programs provided financing of medical care services for persons who, for the most part, were sicker than other population groups and had inadequate financial resources to purchase medical care. It was expected, therefore, that the programs would have two effects on utilization of medical services: first, it would increase the utilization of medical care services by covered persons relative to other persons, and second, utilization of services by covered persons would more closely reflect health status rather than financial or other factors.

As a consequence of these programs, the poor made marked gains in the use of medical services relative to higher income groups during the 1960s. As shown in Table I, physician visits per capita increased uniformly with income in 1964; but by 1969 the very lowest income groups visited physicians more frequently than either middle or higher income groups.

Among the elderly, the uniformly positive relationship between physician visits and income which existed in 1964 was no longer apparent by 1969. Although the use of physician services actually *declined* among the aged poor during the 1960s, their utilization rates increased relative to those of the middle income group and fell relative to that of the upper income group.[4]

Among children, the most dramatic increase in the use of physician services was for those in the middle income group, so that the positive relation between income and utilization was strengthened.

It is noteworthy that, except for children, the middle income group experienced decreased physician visits relative to the lowest income group and absolutely. And, except for the elderly, the upper income group suffered losses relative to the lowest income group and absolutely. The decreased per capita utilization by the upper and middle income groups is too great to be explained solely by the increased use by the poor. While it is hazardous to draw any implications about absolute trends over time based on only three years data for the five-year period, it does suggest the possibility that scarce medical personnel has been rationed—*de facto*—among the many claimants for its services.[5]

For persons covered by Medicare and Medicaid, considerable variation in utilization occurs, counter to that which might be expected on the basis of

TABLE I
PHYSICIAN VISITS PER CAPITA BY AGE AND FAMILY INCOME GROUP,
FISCAL YEARS 1964, 1967, AND CALENDAR YEAR 1969

Age and income group[a]	1964	1967	1969
All ages			
Low income	*4.5*	*4.3*	*4.3*
Middle income	4.3	4.3	4.6
High income	4.5	4.2	4.0
	5.1	4.6	4.3
Ratio, high income to low income	1.19	1.07	.93
Under 15 years			
Low income	2.7	2.8	2.8
Middle income	2.8	3.9	3.6
High income	4.5	4.4	4.3
Ratio, high income to low income	1.67	1.57	1.54
15-64 years			
Low income	4.4	4.6	4.8
Middle income	4.7	4.1	4.1
High income	4.9	4.6	4.2
Ratio, high income to low income	1.11	1.00	.88
65 years and older			
Low income	6.3	5.8	6.1
Middle income	7.0	6.7	5.8
High income	7.3	6.5	7.5
Ratio, high income to low income	1.16	1.12	1.23

Sources: 1964, 1967, Department of Health, Education and Welfare, National Center for Health Statistics, Volume of
Physician Visits by Place of Visit and Type of Service, United States, July 1963-June 1964, Series 10, No. 18
(1965), and issue for July 1966-June 1967, No. 49 (1968); 1969, unpublished tabulations.

(a) Low income is defined as under $4,000 in 1964 and under $5,000 in 1967 and 1969. Middle income is defined as
$4,000-$6,999 in 1964 and $5,000-$9,999 in 1967 and 1969. High income is defined as $7,000 and above in 1964
and $10,000 and above in 1967 and 1969.

differences in "need" for medical care. Differences in utilization by race are
quite marked under both programs, and indicate substantially lower benefits for
blacks than whites. In the Medicare program, higher income persons make the
greatest use of services. Yet both poor and black persons tend to be sicker than
higher income and white persons. Marked geographical differences are also
present in both programs. The following sections summarize some of the most
important disparities.

Medicare

Medicare is a uniform, federal program with the same set of benefits
available to all persons regardless of income, race, or geographical location. Yet,
wide differences exist in the use of services on the basis of each of these factors.
Income is a particularly important determinant of Medicare benefits received by
the elderly. Table II presents data on Medicare supplementary medical insurance
services (including physician services, hospital outpatient services, and home
health services) by various income groups. Three components of Medicare
reimbursements per enrollee are indicated: (1) the percent of all persons enrolled
in the voluntary supplementary medical insurance program who receive services
in excess of the deductible ($50 in 1968); (2) the number of reimbursable
services received by persons exceeding the deductible (reimbursable services are

TABLE II
MEDICARE REIMBURSEMENTS FOR COVERED SERVICES UNDER THE
SUPPLEMENTARY MEDICAL INSURANCE PROGRAM AND PERSONS SERVED,
BY INCOME, 1968

		Supplementary medical insurance services					
	Total	Under $2,000	$2,000-4,999	$5,000-9,999	$10,000-14,999	$15,000 and over	Ratio, highest income to lowest income
Persons receiving reimbursable services per 1000 Medicare enrollees	460.1	438.2	425.9	475.0	527.2	552.3	1.26
Number of reimbursable services per person receiving reimbursable services	26.6	28.7	23.4	26.6	27.5	27.9	.97
Medicare reimbursement per reimbursable service	$7.27	$6.06	$8.11	$8.21	$7.95	$10.40	1.72
Medicare reimbursement per person enrolled	$88.60	$76.32	$80.95	$103.87	$115.10	$160.30	2.10

[1] Including unknown income.

Source: U.S. Department of Health, Education and Welfare, Social Security Administration, Office of Research and Statistics, calculated from unpublished tabulations from the 1968 Current Medical Survey.

counted only after the deductible is exceeded); and (3) the average Medicare payment per reimbursable service.

Medicare Benefits by Income

As shown in Table II, marked disparities in the distribution of medical benefits by income occur in the Medicare program. Medicare reimbursements for medical services per person with income above $15,000 was $160 in 1968, compared with $76 for persons with incomes below $2,000—or more than twice as much for the highest income group as for the lowest. This wide difference in benefits stems from differences in two components of reimbursement—the amounts reimbursed per service and the percent of eligible persons exceeding the deductible.

Average reimbursement per service is 70 percent higher for persons with incomes above $15,000 than for persons with incomes below $2,000. Part of this difference in average reimbursement may be attributable to higher charges for medical services in high income areas. However, part of the difference could reflect higher quality care received by higher income persons or more expensive types of services—such as specialist physician care or in-hospital physician care.

Not only is the average reimbursement per service higher for high income persons exceeding the deductible, a higher proportion of high income persons do, in fact, exceed the $50 deductible. Fifty-five percent of elderly persons with incomes above $15,000 use medical services in excess of the deductible, compared with only 43 percent of persons with incomes below $5,000.

It is interesting to note that the proportion of persons receiving reimbursable services is greater for incomes below $2,000 than for incomes between $2,000 and $5,000. Thereafter, the proportion receiving reimbursable services increases steadily with income. Similarly, persons below $2,000 income exceeding the deductible receive more reimbursable services than persons in the $2,000 to $5,000 income range. Number of services per person then steadily increases with income. The very poorest persons, however, have the lowest average reimbursement per service.

In summary, the strikingly higher level of reimbursement for higher income elderly persons is primarily a reflection of two components—the greater proportion of high income persons who receive services and the higher average payment per service for high income persons. This finding has major implications for the income distributional impact of the Medicare program and for the design of new initiatives in financing medical care services.

First, the supplementary medical insurance plan under the Medicare program is financed by premium payments by elderly persons matched by general revenues. Persons of all income classes pay the same premium, yet higher income persons receive a disproportionate share of benefits. To eliminate this inequitable distribution of net benefits, the premium might be graduated with income or all financing might come from general revenues.

Second, if the Medicare model is to be instructive in the design of national health insurance proposals, it is important to delve more deeply into the basic causes of the disparity in benefits by income class. Several explanations are possible. One explanation that can be quickly discarded is that the pattern simply reflects differences among income groups in "need" for medical care. On virtually any measure of morbidity one cares to select, higher income elderly persons are healthier than lower income elderly persons.

It might be argued that the greater use of physician services under Medicare causes improved health status of high income elderly persons. Although high income persons may purchase preventive care and regular

Health Status of Persons Age 65 or Over, by Income, 1968-69

	Restricted activity days per person per year	Bed disability days per person per year	Percent of persons with some limitation due to chronic conditions
Total[a]			
Family income	*34.3*	*13.7*	*42.4*
Under $3,000	43.0	15.4	50.4
$ 3,000 – 3,999	32.0	13.6	40.9
4,000 – 6,999	28.0	11.5	37.0
7,000 – 9,999	28.7	14.7	37.1
10,000 – 14,999	25.2	11.5	37.2
15,000 and over	23.4	11.7	32.9

Source: U.S. Department of Health, Education and Welfare, National Center for Health Statistics, *Age Patterns in Medical Care, Illness and Disability, United States, 1968-1969,* Series 10, No. 70, Tables 19 and L.

[a]Includes unknown income.

checkups, Medicare does not cover such care. The causation, therefore, does not run from use of Medicare preventive services to better health status. For whatever reason, it appears that healthier elderly persons use more nonpreventive physician services.

The major economic factor which may explain disparity in physician services is the constant coinsurance rate faced by all of the elderly. With the exception of very poor elderly persons covered by Medicaid, all elderly persons must pay the deductible amount ($50 in 1968) and 20 percent of all expenses above that amount. Economic theory predicts that when all persons must pay the same price, higher income persons will use more services (holding constant for other factors such as health status). Therefore, since both a person with $3,000 and a person with $15,000 income must pay 20 percent of all medical expenses above the deductible, that payment will be more of a deterrent to use for the person with $3,000 income. On the other hand, if higher income persons see physicians who charge higher prices without any concomitant increase in real or perceived quality, the greater use of physician services by higher income persons would be partially offset. Higher income persons, however, may be more likely to buy supplementary private insurance to pay the deductible and coinsurance amounts so that the net marginal price to higher income persons is lower.

Moreover, persons in the very lowest income group (family incomes under $2,000) use more physician services than persons with slightly higher incomes ($2,000 to $4,999). This difference could also be a price effect since persons in the very lowest income group are likely to be eligible for Medicaid, and hence pay no deductible or coinsurance charges. However, part of the greater utilization of the very poor may be a consequence of their poorer health status.

If the price effect is a major factor in the differential pattern of use by income class, one way to move toward greater equality in the use of physicians' services would be a financing plan with variable coinsurance and deductible rates depending upon income. The very lowest income groups could face zero or minimal deductible and coinsurance payments while the highest income groups could face more substantial out-of-pocket costs. To simply raise the coinsurance rate from 20 percent to 25 percent for all covered persons, as the Nixon Administration has recently proposed doing in the Medicare program, could be expected to yield even more inequitable patterns of physician use.

In addition to the price effect, other factors may contribute to the differential use of services. Higher income persons tend to be more highly educated, and may place a greater value on medical care generally. Probably even more significant, medical resources are much more abundant in high income areas than in low income areas[6] so that the time, travel, and search costs of obtaining care are lower. Ready availability of medical resources, therefore, may induce a greater use of services for higher income persons. Sorting out the contribution of each of these factors should be a top research priority.

Medicare Benefits by Race

Substantial differences in use of medical services by race also occur in the Medicare program. As shown in Table III, average Medicare reimbursement for physicians' services per enrolled white person was $79 in 1968, compared with $48 for persons of other races—63 percent higher for whites. Most of this difference is attributable to differences in the proportion of eligible persons receiving services, rather than to variations in average payment per person receiving care. Thirty-nine percent of whites enrolled in Medicare received some reimbursable physician services, compared with only 28 percent of persons of other races. Black elderly persons make relatively greater use of hospital outpatient services, but not by an amount sufficient to offset the greater use of private physician services by whites. Medicare reimbursement for both types of services was $81 for white enrollees and $53 for persons of other races.

TABLE III
MEDICARE REIMBURSEMENTS AND PERSONS SERVED, BY RACE, 1968

	Physician Services			Hospital Outpatient Services		
	White	Other races	Ratio white to other races	White	Other races	Ratio white to other races
Persons receiving reimbursable services per 1000 Medicare enrollees	394.9	279.4	1.41	75.7	89:8	.84
Medicare reimbursement per person served	$199.44	$173.37	1.15	$39.02	$50.43	.77
Medicare reimbursement per person enrolled	$78.76	$48.44	1.63	$2.79	$4.53	.62

Source: U.S. Department of Health, Education and Welfare, Social Security Administration, Office of Research and Statistics, *Medicare, 1968: Section 1, Summary*, 1973, Tables 1.11, 1.12, and 1.14.

Again, this disparity in use of services cannot be explained on the basis of health status. Elderly blacks have more restricted activity days, more bed disability days, and more chronic conditions, than elderly whites.[7]

Since elderly blacks tend to be poorer than elderly whites, it might be argued that the same factors which lead to higher utilization by high income elderly persons also contribute to the differential pattern of utilization by race. While 59 percent of elderly whites had incomes below $5,000 in 1970, 78 percent of elderly blacks fell into that income category.[8] Although data are not available from the Medicare program on utilization by race for given income classes, data from the National Center for Health Statistics, Health Interview Survey, indicate that even within a given income class, elderly blacks receive fewer physician services. In fact, high income elderly blacks see the physician less frequently than low income elderly blacks. Lower use by high income blacks might result from better health status and limited availability of physician services to blacks generally.

| Race | Number of physician visits[a] by income and race, age 65 and over, 1969 | | |
	All income[b]	Under $5,000	$5,000 and above
White	6.2	6.2	6.6
Other	5.1	5.5	3.4

Source: U.S. Department of Health, Education and Welfare, National Center for Health Statistics, *Physician Visits, 1969,* Series 10, No. 73, Table 8.

[a]Unlike the Medicare data, these data do not include physician visits to hospital patients.

[b]Includes unknown income.

Unpublished tabulations from the Health Interview Survey also indicate that elderly whites visit physicians more frequently than elderly blacks both in Standard Metropolitan Statistical Areas and in areas outside of major metropolitan areas. Elderly whites with less than a 12th grade education have more physician visits than blacks with similar education; the same relationship is true for persons with more than a 12th grade education.[9]

An explanation for the substantial differential in utilization of physicians' services by race, therefore, must go beyond explanations of inadequate financing (since they exist even within the Medicare program), health status, income, education, or residence. It seems clear there are specific racial barriers to access to medical care. They are perhaps traceable to discrimination on the part of physicians in the types of patients they will treat and the areas in which they will practice to discrimination on the part of medical schools in the types of students admitted. Any financing program applied to all population groups without supplementary measures to increase access to care of minority persons is likely to yield a similarly inequitable pattern of benefits.

Medicare Benefits by Region

Medicare benefits also vary markedly by geographical location (Table IV). Medicare reimbursements for physicians' services per person enrolled, for

TABLE IV
**MEDICARE PHYSICIAN AND OTHER MEDICAL SERVICE REIMBURSEMENTS
AND PERSONS SERVED, BY REGION, 1968**

| | Physicians' Services | | | | |
	U.S.	Northeast	North Central	South	West
Persons receiving physician reimbursable services per 1000 Medicare enrollees	387.8	397.0	358.0	368.6	476.4
Medicare reimbursement for physician services per person served	$198.16	$209.37	$178.01	$192.21	$213.83
Medicare reimbursement for physician services per person enrolled	$76.85	$83.13	$63.73	$71.10	$101.88

Source: U.S. Department of Health, Education and Welfare, Social Security Administration, Office of Research and Statistics, *Medicare, 1968: Section 1, Summary,* 1973, Tables 1.3, 1.5, and 1.6.

example, range from $64 in the North Central region to $102 in the West—or 60 percent higher in the West than in the North Central region. The South region also has quite low reimbursements for physician services—averaging $71 per enrollee in 1968.

Data are available on only two components of average reimbursement per enrollee—the percent of enrollees receiving reimbursable services (services above the deductible amount) and the average reimbursement per person receiving reimbursable services. The patterns by region are quite similar for both components. The percentage of persons receiving physician services ranges from 36 percent in the North Central region to 48 percent in the West (with the South also on the low end of the range at 37 percent).

Variation in reimbursement for physicians' services per person enrolled is not quite as extreme as variation in percentage of enrollees receiving services, but follows a similar regional pattern. Reimbursements per enrollee are 20 percent higher in the West than in the North Central region. This difference could reflect regional price differences. However, if there are systematic differences in number of physician services received per person receiving services by region, these differences would be reflected in the regional pattern.

Data from the Health Interview Survey also confirm that numbers of physician visits vary markedly by region—so that the regional pattern is not just a difference in medical prices. More elderly persons see a physician in the West than in the North Central region, and of those who see a physician, they see the physician more frequently in the West than in the North Central region.

Several explanations of the regional pattern of physician services are possible. First, persons may be healthier in some regions than in others. Second, physicians may be more abundant in some areas than others. In areas with many physicians, the time and travel costs involved in obtaining care may be lower, thus inducing more elderly persons to obtain medical care. In such areas, it may not be necessary for physicians to ration scarce physician time among elderly and non-elderly patients so that with adequate financing more elderly persons obtain care. Or it may be that with an abundance of physicians, physicians

	Percent of elderly persons seeing physician during year	Physician visits per elderly person per year	Physician visits per elderly person seeing physician
All areas	*71.3*	*6.1*	*8.6*
Northeast	72.8	6.5	9.0
North Central	68.8	5.6	8.1
South	71.5	6.0	8.4
West	72.8	6.7	9.3

Source: U.S. Department of Health, Education and Welfare, National Center for Health Statistics, *Age Patterns in Medical Care, Illness, and Disability, United States, 1968-1969,* Series 10, No. 70, Tables 9 and 15.

encourage greater utilization through greater requests for repeat visits.

Data indicate that there is some basis to both of these explanations. Elderly persons in the North Central region do appear to be healthier than elderly persons in the West. Restricted activity days and bed disability days are lower in the North Central region than in the West. Inconsistent with the health status explanation of regional patterns of physician utilization is the high incidence of illness in the South. Restricted activity days, bed disability days, and incidence of chronic conditions are all higher in the South than in any other region, yet elderly persons in the South receive low Medicare reimbursements for physician services.

	Restricted activity days per elderly person per year	Bed disability days per elderly person per year	Percent of elderly persons with some limitation due to chronic conditions
U.S.	*34.3*	*13.7*	*42.4*
Northeast	31.3	13.1	39.4
North Central	30.9	11.4	39.6
South	38.8	16.6	49.5
West	37.3	13.6	38.9

Source: U.S. Department of Health, Education and Welfare, National Center for Health Statistics, *Age Patterns in Medical Care, Illness, and Disability,* U.S. 1968-1969, Series 10, No. 70, Tables 20 and 26.

Explanation of the lower utilization of physician services in the South may lie in the more limited availability of physicians in that region. Both the South and the North Central regions have few patient care physicians per capita (1.01 patient care physicians per 1000 persons in the South and 1.09 in the North Central region).[10] The Northeast and the West have much higher concentrations of physicians (1.99 in the Northeast and 1.43 in the West). Regional patterns in use of physician services, therefore, are quite consistent with regional patterns in numbers of physicians per capita.

Before leaving the evidence on regional patterns of physician utilization under the Medicare program, it is instructive to return to the racial disparities in the Medicare program presented above. It might be argued that the greater use of physician services by whites is a reflection of regional differences. In particular, since elderly persons of other races are disproportionately represented in the South (60 percent of elderly persons of other races live in the South compared with 26 percent of elderly whites), part of the racial difference may simply be a reflection of lower utilization by persons in the South generally.

Table V presents data on reimbursements for physicians' services and persons receiving services by race within regions. As shown in the table, substantial racial differences exist within each region. In the North Central region, Medicare reimbursements per person enrolled are 24 percent higher for

TABLE V

MEDICARE PHYSICIAN AND OTHER MEDICAL SERVICES, PERSONS SERVED
AND AVERAGE REIMBURSEMENTS, BY REGION AND RACE, 1968

	White	Other races	Ratio, white to other races
	Persons served per 1,000 enrollees		
All areas	*394.9*	*279.4*	*1.413*
Northeast	400.4	326.3	1.227
North Central	361.5	305.6	1.183
South	391.9	241.5	1.623
West	478.7	437.1	1.095
	Reimbursement per person served		
All areas	*$199.44*	*$173.37*	*1.150*
Northeast	209.91	196.82	1.067
North Central	178.27	169.71	1.050
South	195.96	163.07	1.202
West	214.86	183.42	1.171
	Reimbursement per person enrolled		
All areas	*$78.76*	*$48.44*	*1.626*
Northeast	84.05	64.22	1.309
North Central	64.44	51.85	1.243
South	76.80	39.37	1.951
West	102.86	80.17	1.283

Source: Unpublished tabulations from 1968 Medicare Summary based on bills for reimbursed services for a 5 percent sample of the enrolled population; Office of Research and Statistics, Social Security Administration, U.S. Department of Health, Education and Welfare.

whites than for persons of other races. The South has by far the most extreme racial disparity, with elderly whites receiving 95 percent higher physician reimbursements per person enrolled than elderly persons of other races. Discriminatory practices, particularly in the South, would again appear to be the basic explanation for differences in Medicare benefits by race.

Medicaid

Unlike the Medicare program, the Medicaid program is a federal-state program in which individual states have substantial leeway in setting eligibility standards, and comprehensiveness of benefits. In spite of more generous federal matching for low income states, high income states receive a disproportionate share of Medicaid benefits. This causes a poor matching between poor persons and Medicaid funds. Forty-six percent of poor persons live in the South, but only 17 percent of Medicaid benefits go to that region.[11]

While geographical variation in benefits might be expected from the nature of the Medicaid program, somewhat more significant is the distribution of benefits by race. Twenty-four states reported Medicaid payments and recipients by race in 1969. Only two states from the Northeast region, New York and Connecticut, reported such data. Several states with large Medicaid programs, including Massachusetts and California, did not submit data by race. No state in the Pacific region with a Medicaid program supplied breakdowns by race. There is no assurance, therefore, that available data are representative of the entire Medicaid program.

Meaningful comparisons are further limited by absence of data on eligible Medicaid persons. Data reported are based on recipients of any Medicaid services. States which make an effort to provide at least some medical services to nearly all eligible persons could be expected to have fairly low payments per recipient while states restricting benefits to a few, seriously ill persons would have high average payments per recipient.

Information is based on a full year's data, but not all Medicaid recipients are eligible for services for the entire year. Variations among states or population groups in the average length of time covered by Medicaid could distort comparisons.

Medicaid Benefits by Race

On the basis of reported data, differences in Medicaid benefits by race are even greater than under the Medicare program. Including all types of medical services (as well as hospital and nursing home care), average Medicaid payments per white recipient of services was $375 in 1969, compared with only $213 for other races. As shown in Table VI, whites receive higher Medicaid payments per recipient of service in every geographical region, and in every age group. Differences among the elderly are particularly wide, with elderly whites averaging $696 compared with $328 for elderly persons of other races. Only for children in some geographical areas, such as cities with 400,000 or more population, do racial differences disappear.

TABLE VI
**MEDICAID PAYMENTS FOR ALL MEDICAL SERVICES PER RECIPIENT,
BY RACE, AGE, REGION, AND RESIDENCE, 1969[1]**

	All ages		Under 21		21-64		65 and Over	
	White	Other Races	White	Other Races	White	Other Races	White	Other Races
All areas	$375.44	$212.85	$130.10	$116.80	$446.77	$340.63	$696.09	$328.08
Region								
Northeast	361.87	204.73	131.72	120.25	421.21	303.26	981.88	400.98
North Central	448.52	249.46	135.48	121.52	575.85	441.68	730.51	452.90
South	322.39	180.18	116.82	102.03	387.42	289.12	412.85	208.62
Mountain	302.59	213.12	100.27	116.94	383.53	361.79	586.70	416.51
Residence								
City, 400,000 or more population	332.80	221.34	122.20	125.54	381.38	354.97	763.33	399.99
Other SMSA	425.96	227.54	141.44	113.60	531.78	376.13	678.50	351.31
Non-SMSA	406.10	178.57	135.95	86.11	524.97	274.95	660.26	232.55

[1]Based on data from 24 states with Medicaid programs in 1969 and reporting data by race.

Source: Calculated from unpublished State Medicaid reports, U.S. Department of Health, Education and Welfare, National Center for Social Statistics.

Disparities in benefits by race are not quite as marked for physicians' services as for *all* medical services. As shown in Table VII, whites receiving any Medicaid services average physician payments of $35 compared with $25 for other races. Most of this difference is accounted for by the higher percentage of

TABLE VII
MEDICAID PHYSICIAN SERVICES, BY RACE AND AGE, 1969[1]

	Physician payments per Medicaid recipient		Physician payments per visit		Physician visits for persons seeing physician		Persons seeing physician per 1,000 Medicaid recipients	
	White	Other Races	White	Other Races	White	Other Races	White	Other Races
Total	$35.29	$25.53	$ 9.23	$ 9.19	6.36	5.41	602	514
By Age								
Under 21	24.20	17.63	11.86	10.70	3.40	3.28	599	503
21-64	51.75	39.67	12.97	11.27	6.98	6.71	572	524
65 and Over	34.00	26.81	5.16	4.56	10.26	10.85	642	542

[1]Based on data from 23 states with Medicaid programs in 1969 and reporting data by race.

Source: Calculated from unpublished state Medicaid reports, U.S. Department of Health, Education and Welfare, National Center for Social Statistics.

white Medicaid recipients who use physician services. Only 52 percent of persons of other races who receive any Medicaid services also receive physicians' services compared with 60 percent of whites. Physician visits per person for those who see a physician range from 6.4 for whites to 5.4 for other races. In part, however, this is attributable to the greater predominance of children (who average fewer visits than older persons) among the recipients of other races. Fewer elderly persons of other races see a physician, but those who visit a physician do so more frequently.

Because of the limitations of the data, evidence from additional sources should be examined before drawing any definitive conclusions about the distribution of Medicaid benefits by race. The pattern observed in the Medicaid program, however, underscores a similar distribution of benefits by race in the Medicare program, and may well be indicative of racial barriers to care for poor persons as well as elderly persons.

ACCESS TO MEDICAL CARE AND DESIGN OF FINANCING PROGRAMS

Experience with the Medicare program has been belabored at some length in this paper because it is the major experience we have had with a uniform financing program. It is always possible that the experience of the elderly is not generally applicable to other age groups. Younger persons may be more able and more willing to seek out medical care over a wider geographical area—so that differences among communities in availability of medical manpower do not lead to extreme differences in utilization of medical services. Elderly persons of other races may be more restrained in seeking medical care than younger persons as a result of years and years of discriminatory practices that may no longer be as widespread.

Offsetting these arguments, however, is evidence that the same type of patterns found for the elderly under Medicare exist for persons of all age groups. For every income class, white persons of every age group typically see the physician more frequently than persons of other races. For every type of residence, white persons of every age group typically see the physician more frequently than persons of other races.[12] It seems likely that if a program such as Medicare were to cover the non-elderly as well, many of the same disparities would occur.

Since the Medicare program is the only one of its kind, experience with this program cannot be lightly dismissed, and its lessons for design of national health insurance covering all persons cannot be ignored. A financing plan which guarantees "equal financial access" to medical care cannot be relied upon to yield equal access for persons of all incomes, races, and geographical areas. Instead, such a program is likely to systematically favor high income persons, white persons, and persons in areas with an abundance of medical resources.

If greater equality in the use of medical services, or an increase in utilization of services by those persons with lower levels of utilization, is desired, two possible types of approaches might be taken. First, uniform financing plans might be supplemented with direct policies to reduce nonfinancial barriers to access. For example, the supply of medical manpower and facilities might be increased in low-income areas, in minority neighborhoods, and in geographical regions with low utilization. By so doing, the time, transportation, and search costs involved in obtaining medical care could be reduced. Educational programs could be conducted to help overcome patient attitudes which restrict access to care. Existing regulations on discriminatory practices could be more vigorously enforced and applied to all providers of medical services receiving payments under public programs.

A second type of approach would be to structure a financing program in such a way as to help overcome both financial and nonfinancial barriers to access. Clearly, to attempt to design a financing plan which would completely offset existing patterns of distribution of medical resources and discriminatory practices is an impossible task, and undoubtedly not the most efficient, even if feasible, method of achieving social goals. But to forfeit the possibility of structuring the financing plan in such a way as to help offset nonfinancial barriers to access seems to be equally absurd. Causing massive changes in the existing distribution of medical resources promises to be a slow, costly, and perhaps impossible task as well. In any event it seems unlikely that resources currently residing in high income areas can be induced to move to other locations. New direct policies, therefore, will have to be directed at increasing the supply of medical resources in low-income and minority neighborhoods, rather than diverting existing resources away from high income areas. Such a procedure is quite slow, and costly in terms of the proportion of society's resources which will be required for medical care.

It seems worthwhile, therefore, to explore the possibility of designing a financing plan which provides not "equal financial access" but one which systematically favors those groups which face barriers to access on other grounds. The following sections develop how such a plan might be devised.

Reducing Inequality of Utilization by Income

One of the sources of inequality in utilization of medical services, which is easiest to attack with a financing program, is that caused by income differences. Specifically; if the poor are required to pay lower prices for medical services than the rich, some of the income effect can be offset. Making the rich pay higher prices by such means as taxing their medical care consumption is unlikely to be a politically attractive scheme, but tapering off the benefits of a public financing plan as income rises is a less controversial, and probably politically feasible, alternative.

Several income-related benefit plans have been proposed. Pauly designed a variable subsidy coinsurance plan for low-income persons, and Feldstein advocated a more general income-related benefit plan for persons of all incomes. More recently, a staff paper in the U.S. Department of Health, Education and Welfare, has designed an illustrative income-related plan called the Maximum Liability Health Insurance Plan.[13] All of these plans have the characteristic that the lowest income persons pay the lowest fraction of medical expenses as a result of fairly low coinsurance and deductible provisions. As income increases, the patient's portion of the bill is increased.

Neglecting for the moment differences in physical access and attitudinal barriers to access, Figure 1 illustrates how a varying schedule of out-of-pocket payments can increase utilization by low-income persons. As economic theory predicts, higher prices are shown to reduce utilization of medical services while, for a given price, utilization increases with income. A person with income of Y_1 who faces a price of $\overline{p}$ will demand X_1 units of medical care, or less than the "acceptable" level of care (however defined) X_a. An individual with a somewhat higher income Y_2, who faces the same price will demand X_2 units of medical care, only somewhat below the "acceptable" level. An individual with income Y_3 who faces the same price will demand X_3 units of medical care, or more than the "acceptable" level.

If instead of having all persons pay the same price, no charges were levied for persons with incomes of Y_1, those individuals would demand X_a, the "acceptable" level of care as the figure is drawn. Similarly, persons with incomes of Y_2 could be induced to demand X_a units of medical care if they were required to pay only half of the price.

What would happen if no direct charges at all were levied on individuals? Would "equal financial" access for all persons lead to equal utilization? If there were no systematic differences in physical access or attitudes of patients and physicians in relation to income, equal utilization might reasonably be expected to occur for all persons of a given health status. This *if* turns out to be a very big *if*. In fact, medical resources are much more abundant in high income areas so that the time involved in obtaining care and the transportation and search costs are substantially lower for higher income persons than lower income persons.[14] Furthermore, physicians may well have a preference for treating persons of their own socioeconomic class (characterized by high income among other things),

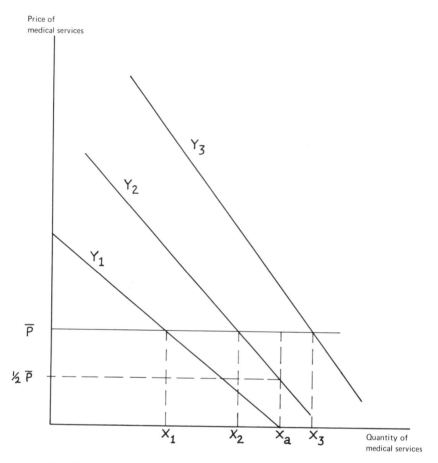

Figure 1. Demand for medical care for different income
levels $(Y_3 > Y_2 > Y_1)$ for a given health status

and for a given remuneration will be willing to supply a smaller quantity of
services to lower income persons than to higher income persons. In addition,
education tends to be systematically related to income so that higher income
persons may have a stronger recognition of the benefits of medical care and,
hence, seek medical care more readily. It seems unlikely, therefore, that zero
direct charges on medical care will result in equal utilization by income.

A great many difficulties are involved in implementing an income-related
national health insurance plan. Some estimate must be made about the set of
relative price subsidies which will induce that degree of equality in utilization of
medical services which is desired (or will bring lower income persons up to the
desired level of utilization). A final decision on a desirable schedule of
income-related benefits would also hinge on cost considerations—how much

society is willing to invest in achieving this particular social goal (perhaps at the expense of other desirable social goals). Given the noted failure of uniform financing programs to achieve much equality in use of medical services, however, such a plan seems worthy of consideration.

Physical Access and Unequal Utilization

The claim is frequently made that it does no good to pay for medical services if those services are not available. While on the face of it, this claim seems sensible enough, medical services are, in fact, available to most persons somewhere at some cost. If the resources are not available in the immediate vicinity, time, travel, and search costs incurred in obtaining care might be quite substantial—but with enough financial inducement, it should be feasible to overcome these barriers to access.

Figure 2 illustrates the demand for medical services given monetary and nonmonetary costs of care including time, travel, and search costs as well as price of medical care. If the same price for medical care is faced by all persons, but the time, travel, and transportation cost is higher for low income persons, lower income persons will utilize fewer services (again, holding health status constant). As shown in Figure 2a, a person with income of Y_1, who pays a price for medical care of p_0 and faces other costs of t_1 will demand X_1 units of medical care. Higher income persons paying the same price for medical care but facing lower other costs will demand greater quantities. However, utilization of lower income persons can be increased by lowering the price of medical care. As shown in Figure 2b, if the price paid for medical care for a person with income of Y_1 is reduced from p_0 to p_1 (which may be zero), the quantity of medical care demanded will increase to the acceptable level. Similarly, reducing the price of medical care to a person with income of Y_2 from p_0 to p_2 (which is still somewhat higher than the p_1 faced by a lower income person) will also increase the quantity demanded up to the acceptable level.

Therefore, by picking an appropriate set of price subsidies, it is possible to overcome physical barriers to access for low-income persons by reducing the monetary costs of care. For some very poor persons, it is possible that the time, travel, and search costs of obtaining care are so high that even at a zero price for medical care, they will still demand a lower than acceptable level. In this case it may be necessary for the financing plan to pay transportation costs as well as medical care.

Racial Barriers to Access

Financing plans seem less capable of overcoming racial barriers to access than those related to income or location. While it would be possible to design a higher schedule of coinsurance rates for whites than for members of other races, such a proposal is unlikely to have substantial political appeal.

It seems imperative that specific supply programs to increase access of minorities be conducted if any significant impact on racial disparities in public

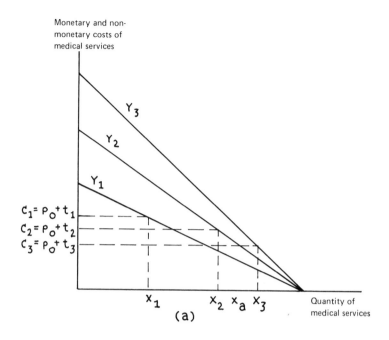

$$c_1 = p_0 + t_1$$
$$c_2 = p_0 + t_2$$
$$c_3 = p_0 + t_3$$

(a)

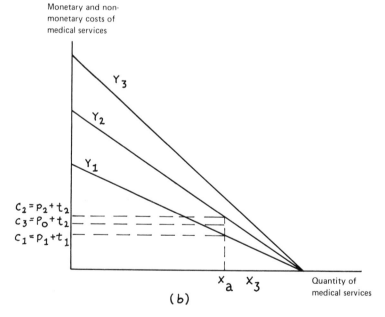

$$c_2 = p_2 + t_2$$
$$c_3 = p_0 + t_2$$
$$c_1 = p_1 + t_1$$

(b)

Figure 2. Demand for medical care for different income levels
($Y_3 > Y_2 > Y_1$) with different physical access ($t_1 > t_2 > t_3$)

financing programs is to be made. Subsidies to minority students to attend medical school, training minority residents as paramedical personnel, expansion of hospital outpatient facilities in central cities, are all possible methods of attacking this problem.

Even with an adequate national health insurance financing plan, it might be desirable to continue providing operating subsidies to organizations which locate in minority neighborhoods—such as neighborhood health centers and health maintenance organizations. Selective use of such subsidies could further reduce the cost of medical care to minority members, and help achieve a greater equality among races in access to medical services.

CONCLUSION

This chapter has had two objectives: (1) reviewing the impact of existing financing programs on use of medical care services, particularly physicians' services; and (2) outlining how a financing program might be designed to overcome barriers to access to medical care.

The major finding of the paper has been the disparity in utilization of physicians' services among income, racial, and geographical groups—even with a uniform financing plan such as Medicare. Under Medicare, persons with incomes above $15,000 receive reimbursement for physicians' services twice that of persons with incomes below $5,000. Reimbursements for physician services are 63 percent higher for elderly whites than for persons of other races. Elderly persons in the West receive payments 60 percent above that received by elderly persons in the North Central region. Geographical and racial disparities are also present in the Medicaid program, with white recipients receiving payments for all medical services 76 percent above that received by Medicaid recipients of other races.

The review of existing financing programs, primarily Medicare, has focused on physicians' services in an attempt to infer indirectly the impact of financing programs on access to primary care. Unfortunately, data on primary care are not directly available from existing programs. Restricting attention to physicians' services omits from consideration other providers of primary care services—such as public health nurses. Perhaps more importantly, physicians' services include both primary care services and specialized services. Patterns of utilization of primary care services, therefore, may be substantially different from that of all physicians' services.

It seems likely, however, that the disparities among income, racial, and geographical groups which exist for all physicians' services are even more extreme for primary care services. When medical conditions deteriorate to the point of requiring specialized care, normal barriers to access are likely to be overcome. Persons will be willing to travel longer distances and use savings or incur debt for treatment of conditions which are life-threatening or extremely painful. Preventive services or early treatment of illness are more likely to be neglected if financial, physical, or attitudinal barriers are present. Therefore, while a definitive estimate of the effect of financing programs on access to primary care cannot be made with existing data, it seems safe to conclude that even with uniform financing programs, substantial disparities in access to primary care occur with respect to income, race, and geographical location.

Experience with the Medicare program makes it clear that assuring "equal financial access" to medical care for all persons will not result in equal access for persons of all incomes, races, and geographical areas. Instead, such a program is likely to systematically favor high income persons, white persons, and persons in areas with an abundance of medical resources. If greater equality in the use of medical services, or an increase in utilization of services by those persons with lower levels of utilization, is desired, two approaches show promise. First, a financing plan should be designed which provides not "equal financial access" but one which systematically favors those groups which face barriers to access on other grounds. An income-related national health insurance plan is one such approach. Second, direct supply programs should be pursued to supplement such a financing plan, with particular emphasis on increasing access to medical care of minority groups.

REFERENCES

1. For a discussion of the goal of equal access, see Linday, C. M., Medical Care and the Economics of Sharing, *Economica,* 36, No. 144, 351-62, November, 1969; and Garfinkel, I., Equal Access, Minimum Provision, and Efficiency in Financing Medical Care, *Journal of Human Resources,* 7, No. 2, 242-49, Spring 1972. For an overall discussion of the issue of financing to achieve access to care see Fein, R., On Achieving Access and Equity in Health Care, in Andreopoulos, S. (Ed.), MEDICAL CURE AND MEDICAL CARE, *Milbank Memorial Fund Quarterly,* Vol. L, No. 4, pp. 157-90, October, 1972 (Part 2).

2. See information submitted by Office of Management and Budget in response to requests from the Joint Economic Committee, March, 1973, p. 11.

3. Including altruistic benefits makes this definition of acceptable care somewhat circular. Altruistic benefits may be related to pervading views about medical necessity and prevailing standards of utilization. However, rather than having a single point at which care is unacceptable or acceptable, altruistic benefits presumably decline gradually with additional care.

4. Lowenstein also finds a decline in physician visits by the elderly after Medicare. (See Lowenstein, R., Early Effects of Medicare on Health Care of the Aged, *Social Security Bulletin,* 34, No. 4, 3-20.

5. Data from 1970 currently available by age group indicate substantial increases in physician visits from 1969 to 1970. Average visits increased from 4.3 for all age groups in 1969 to 4.6 in 1970. National Center for Health Statistics, Current Estimates, 1970, Series 10, No. 72.

6. "In 1970 the 15 counties with the highest per capita incomes had seven times as many patient care physicians per capita as did the 15 counties with the lowest per capita incomes, 26 times as many physician specialsts per capita, and three times as many hospital beds per capita." Davis, K., Health Insurance, in Schultze, C. L., et al., SETTING NATIONAL PRIORITIES: THE 1973 BUDGET, The Brookings Institution, Washington, D.C., p. 222.

7. For comparison of health status of elderly whites and elderly persons of other races, see Davis, K., Financial Medical Care Services: the Federal Role, in HEARINGS ON THE COSTS OF MEDICAL CARE, Subcommittee on Consumer Economics, Joint Economic Committee, forthcoming.

8. Calculated from Current Population Reports, Consumer Income, U.S. Department of Commerce, Bureau of the Census, Characteristics of the Low-Income Population 1970, Series P-60, No. 81, November, 1971.

9. See unpublished tabulations from the 1969 Health Interview Survey reported in Wilensky, G. R., Utilization of Ambulatory Care, Urban Institute Working Paper, 963-3.

10. American Medical Association, Distribution of Physicians in the United States, Chicago, Illinois, 1970.

11. See Davis, K., Financing Medical Care Services: The Federal Role.

12. See unpublished tabulations from the Health Interview Survey published in Wilensky, *op. cit.*

13. Pauly, M. V., An Analysis of Government Health Insurance Plans for Poor Families, *Public Policy,* 19, No. 3 (Summer 1971, pp. 489-521); Feldstein, M. S., A New Approach to National Health Insurance, *Public Interest,* No. 23 (Spring 1971, pp. 93-105; and Comprehensive HEW Simplification and Reform, Mega Proposal, Hearings Before the Committee on Labor and Public Welfare, U.S. Senate, 1973.

14. It is sometimes argued that higher income persons have higher time costs since their wages are higher. This is true only for working high income persons—and would not apply to high income wives who do not work (and who could better afford babysitters to watch children while obtaining medical care themselves). Even for high income persons who work, such persons are more likely to have generous sick leave provisions than low income persons and are not likely to be docked pay for time spent obtaining medical care.

ACKNOWLEDGMENT

The author, a research associate with The Brookings Institution, wishes to thank Duran Bell, Jr., for helpful comments. The views presented here are those of the author and not necessarily those of the officers, trustees or other staff members of The Brookings Institution.

DISCUSSION

DANIEL O. WAGSTER: I want to congratulate Dr. Davis on the scholarly and provocative paper. She exhibited remarkable discipline in restricting herself to a purely economist's point of view. In her attempt to make available to us a series of theoretical possibilities, she has not been constrained by operational viewpoints, political uncertainties or management conservatism. At the same time the paper recognizes the importance of *money* in health care delivery, i.e., money in terms of prices as well as implicit costs such as time, travel, and education. This recognition of money is in contrast to the currently popular position in some important places that modern medical care does not really need money to provide quality care.

I cannot resist the temptation to remind you of a basic deficiency in the group practice prepaid plans in terms of the reimbursement arrangement with the Social Security Administration for Medicare beneficiaries. The basis of payment is *cost only,* which means that Medicare recipients are subsidized by those under 65 as to capital requirements. Yet, if these plans (now predominantly called health maintenance organizations) are to keep pace with the standard of care in the community, they must continue to spend capital for new and replacement equipment and facilities at a rate which exceeds allowable depreciation reimbursement from the Social Security Administration. This limitation applies to other Part A providers, but it is especially onerous to hospital-based group practice plans whose membership and facility requirements are expanding.

Unhappily, it is easy to agree Medicare and Medicaid have contributed to inflation, as Dr. Davis points out. The method of financing has reduced the financial burden of certain population segments, thereby increasing the demand and expectation without increasing the supply. There are no incentives to change the delivery system. In fact, there are dis-incentives as in the case cited above in which the Social Security Administration refuses to accept a capital requirement factor in HMO reimbursement. Even though some plans have offered to accept the risk for Medicare beneficiaries on a prospective capitation basis, this legislative and regulatory precedent is of great concern in any discussion of financing methods for health care. For possibly different reasons than Dr. Davis suggests, I agree with her statement that the Medicare "lessons for design on national health insurance covering all persons cannot be ignored."

Dr. Davis did accept the constraint of an artificial segmentation of the spectrum of medical services, i.e., the separation of *primary care* as opposed to secondary which, in turn, is distinct from tertiary care. As you know, hospital based group practice plans are committed to integrated care with continuity of comprehensive services. These embrace preventive, ambulatory, inpatient care, general practitioner, specialist care, diagnostic procedures and so on, irrespective of entry point. It is difficult to visualize the natural division of "primary care" from the spectrum of medical services, and there is reason for some reflection as to the implications of making primary care a distinct segment.

There is a lesson in history which may apply here. The private insurance approach, which gave prepayment its start, covered *inpatient medical services* only and it has taken many years for consumers and providers to make meaningful progress toward overcoming that deficiency. Could the pendulum be swinging too far in another direction when the attempt is being made to separate out and emphasize the "primary care" portion of needed medical services? Should we compartmentalize primary care?

Without rendering judgment on the validity of the economic theory involved in Dr. Davis's paper, there are some aspects which seem to need clarification:

1. Medical services are lumped together in the statistics used. Does this mark important information?

2. Might not income be a proxy variable for race, education, geographic residence, etc.? Should the variables be studied independently before a conclusion is reached?

3. Is the price of medical services the primary barrier to access and does manipulating the price produce a one-for-one effect on demand?

4. If price, variable coinsurance or both are among determinants of demand for medical services, how would a national program deal with high income people buying additional insurance to fill the gaps?

5. Is access the same as utilization or is there an aspect of consumer perception involved?

6. Is the middle class problem of access solved by financing either an

income-related national health insurance plan or direct supply programs that emphasize increasing access of minority groups to medical care?

In conclusion, I would like to comment on three items concerning financing medical care and access to care. In deference to Dr. Davis, I would put these considerations in the manager's corner, not the economist's.

First, the federal financing mechanism (the paper assumed the word *federal*) must be concerned about the organization and delivery of medical care. On the positive side, the financing mechanism would offer incentives to help pull providers and other parties together despite the fact they have not adopted partnership modes in the face of opportunity to do so for over a generation. It is apparent that until recently it has been in each provider's self interest to remain independent. On the negative side, the federal role should avoid affecting adversely organizations considered to have value.

Second, there is need to have a financing mechanism that assures quality, in addition to having an over-riding concern about costs. Some measures for assuring quality in medical services are needed, and the sooner they are developed the better.

Third, the financing mechanism must be flexible enough to allow a pluralistic system of health care services to continue. It is conceivable that a federal financing mechanism could threaten the survival of group practice prepayment plans as they exist today.

IV CONCLUSIONS AND
RECOMMENDATIONS

Primary Care as a Part of the Personal Health Care System

Report of a Symposium

Health care is a pressing social and political issue in the United States. Proposals for change in the organization, financing and provision of personal health services are being made with increasing force and frequency.

The Sun Valley Forum on National Health, a nonprofit institution, was established in 1971 to pursue educational activities concerning various aspects of the nation's health care system. In June 1971, the Forum addressed a major symposium to the financing of the nation's health care system. In June 1972, the Forum turned to the question of the organization of the nation's system for delivering medical care. This year's symposium was devoted to a critical segment of the health field—the provision of primary health care.

The 1973 symposium of the Forum commissioned four leading experts in health care services to prepare and present papers on key sub-topics to the symposium participants. The 31 participants in the symposium (listed at the beginning of this book) included practicing physicians from urban and rural areas, academicians, medical care specialists, economists, administrators, government officials, members of the press, lawyers, and insurance and health care industry executives.

At the close of the 1973 symposium, the participants reviewed this Report. No one was asked to sign the Report, and it should not be assumed that any participant necessarily subscribes to every conclusion appearing in it. But except where the Report indicates that a participant accepted the opportunity to dissent or to express a separate opinion, the Report represents the sense of the Symposium.

PRIMARY HEALTH CARE

I.   Primary Health Care as a Part of the Personal Health Care System

1. Health care in the United States is changing rapidly. Many families feel this change most directly when they cannot find a traditional family physician, when they cannot obtain medical assistance at night, when they cannot pay their medical bills, when they cannot find the quality and scope of health care they require.

2. A useful approach to understanding the problems of the health care system is to focus separately on several levels of personal health care: the primary, secondary and tertiary levels. Very roughly, *primary care* can be said to be the range of services traditionally provided by the general practitioner; *secondary care* refers to the cluster of services provided by the specialist and the inpatient part of the local hospital; *tertiary care* refers to the highly specialized services of the larger medical centers, usually connected to a medical school. These categories are imprecise and overlapping, but are adequate to focus discussion. It must be emphasized, however, that the fact primary care can be considered and discussed separately does not mean that it should be *provided* separately; in fact, the successful delivery of primary care can only be accomplished if it is integrated into the total health care system.

3. The area of primary care is the all-important contact point between the individual and the health care system. The traditional system of primary care was based on the family practitioner who, at his best, knew his patients over a lifetime as well as their families and community. He administered medical care, and also advice. The poor and minority groups, however, were largely outside this system and were generally sent to charity hospitals.

This traditional system appears to be breaking down for a number of reasons:

(a) Most physicians educated after World War II do not want to be general practitioners in the traditional mode.
(i)   The working conditions are often considered too onerous;
(ii) The changing nature of medical education, away from apprenticeship with a practicing physician and toward residency at a hospital, has substantially eliminated an important entry point for the young physician into primary care.
(iii) The medical schools and the profession generally emphasize specialization and the higher status of practicing specialty medicine.
(b) The high mobility of our population and the trend toward urban living have broken down traditional relationships between the physician and his patients.
(c) The complexities of modern primary care make it nearly impossible for one person practicing independently to do a totally adequate task, and organizational substitutes for the solo practitioners have not

developed rapidly enough.

(d) Minority groups and the poor are demanding adequate medical care, and their special needs require the development of new arrangements to provide health care to these groups.

Although statistics are neither complete nor conclusive, it would appear on the basis of 1969 figures that private practitioners still provide about 77 percent of primary care; hospitals provide 12 percent through outpatient clinics and 7 percent through emergency rooms; and the remaining 4 percent is divided among prepaid group practice (3.6 percent), neighborhood health centers, free clinics, and similar institutions.

4. An important cause for concern about our health care system today is that cost levels of medical care of all kinds—including primary care—have skyrocketed in the last seven years.

5. Dissatisfaction with the present system of primary care is substantial, especially among special categories of consumers.

(a) *Inner city residents* have a particularly difficult problem gaining access to primary care. For example, available statistics indicate there is a lower utilization of health care by blacks than the general population even at equal income and educational levels. Inner city residents face particular problems in terms of availability, since few doctors reside or maintain offices in these areas (although this factor is occasionally offset by the availability of hospitals and other health programs). They face social and cultural barriers ranging from outright discrimination to financial impediments and transportation difficulties. Also, it would appear that the quality of health care received by inner-city residents, the continuity of their service and the general support and educative services they receive are of a lower standard than that of the population generally.

(b) *Non-English speaking groups* generally suffer the disabilities of the inner-city population with the added handicap of linguistic barriers that require not only translators and foreign language health providers but also increased attention to cultural factors.

(c) *The poor and working poor* suffer obvious financial and non-financial barriers to the use of health care facilities; they experience more illness and have less access to acceptable primary care services. Fairness in the financing system is a particular problem in relation to families with low income. Because of inequities in the Medicaid system, the working poor are often required to bear the full cost of health care while families on welfare with almost identical incomes appear to receive substantial governmental assistance in meeting these expenses.

(d) *Rural populations* have been faced with a marked decline in the number of physicians serving their primary care needs. This trend has been caused in part by general social attitudes that have attracted highly trained people into urban areas, and in part by specific factors relating to the medical profession—the emphasis in the medical schools on specialties which require large institutions and large population groups, and also the failure of financial incentives to affect significantly the geographic distribution of physicians. Because secondary level health care is often not readily available in rural areas, the scope of primary care must actually be greater than in urban areas.

(e) *The elderly* have the most frequent need for health services. Under present circumstances they often rely too heavily on institutional care—secondary care—because primary care is not available to them. The elderly often face heavy financial burdens even with Medicare as well as other barriers such as transportation difficulties.

6. The major priorities in improved primary care should be directed to improving access and the range and quality of services to the groups described in the preceding paragraph. Also important, however, are the problems facing working and middle class families, for these groups also face a primary care system that is often unsatisfactory. Access for them is usually less of a problem than the special groups described above, but even advantaged groups often find the services provided impersonal and fragmented, not functioning at night and on weekends, expensive, and inadequate in terms of quality and scope of service.

7. Many scholarly observers, government officials, hospital administrators, and other professional health service providers have become conscious of what they perceive to be inefficiencies in the present arrangements, which lead to inflated costs, misallocation of skills and constriction of potentially available outputs of health care.

8. Although all aspects of health care require improvement, the *primary care system* should be given special attention and high priority at this time by educators, practitioners, health administrators and policymakers, for the following reasons:

(a) This is the level of health care delivery comprising the vast majority of basic health services actually delivered and is the area of great dissatisfaction by many consumers.

(b) A poorly functioning primary care system often has the effect of denying access to needed health care at other levels.

(c) The primary care providers interact most directly with other aspects of social and community life, such as the public health, education, environmental concerns, which are increasingly recognized as having an important bearing on health maintenance.

(d) While pervasive in its impact, primary care does not generally have high status associated with secondary and tertiary institutions (hospitals and medical schools), and therefore its problems have tended in the recent past to be ignored or minimized. Hardware, biomedical research and specialization, while important, have received disproportionate attention in recent years, causing the balance between primary care on the one hand, and secondary and tertiary care on the other, to become distorted.

(e) Patterns of delivering primary care are beginning to undergo change from the single practitioner to more complex organizations. This is a propitious time to influence the development of the system—before new fractionated structures become established and resistant to change.

(f) In a period of rapid escalation of the costs of health care, increased attention to primary care may provide one of the most efficient methods to utilize the additional resources which through public and private means will be channeled into the health care field.

II. Design for a Better Primary Care System

9. The field of health care has not developed adequate standards for measuring the quality of service. The development of such standards, in measurable terms where possible, should be a matter of high priority, for it affects all areas of policy making relating to health care.

10. At its best, a fully developed primary care system would perform the following functions:

(a) It would provide an entry, screening and referral point for the rest of the health care system.

(b) It would seek not only to cure or alleviate specific complaints, but also to assume responsibility for health maintenance, i.e., to preserve health, prevent disease, assist the chronically ill and care for common illnesses and disabilities.

(c) It would be concerned with human support services which are necessary for the effective utilization of the health care system, such as essential transportation or home visits and the often neglected function of educating consumers to basic health practices.

(d) It would serve as a focal point for coordinating and monitoring the various health services that a patient may require by referring him to specialists and hospitals and by following through on his later recuperative care.

11. The following general criteria can be used to evaluate the adequacy of primary care in general, and the various types of organizations presently within that system:

(a) *Elimination of barriers to access.* There are serious impediments to access to primary care by one or more barriers, of which the following are the most important:

(i) *Availability.* A prerequisite to access to primary care is the availability of a primary care provider. Availability is a serious problem in many rural areas and, together with other factors such as poverty, poor education, inadequate transportation and patterns of discrimination, is also a problem in many inner-city areas.

(ii) *Location.* The location of many health care facilities, combined with difficulties of transportation, often discourage use of the health care system.

(iii) *Social, cultural and linguistic factors.* Many groups in society, minority and poverty groups in particular, often exhibit behavior patterns that do not result in optimal use of health services. These behavior patterns are rooted in social, cultural and psychological characteristics, which must be recognized and understood if effective health care is to be provided.

(iv) *Inconvenient hours of service.* Working people, for example, often cannot take advantage of a health care provider whose office hours are only 9 a.m. to 5 p.m. on weekdays.

(v) *Financial barriers.* While financial cost affects all aspects of health care, it probably discourages primary care more than secondary treatment, since the illnesses or disabilities dealt with on the primary level are usually easier to neglect.

(b) *More equal use of service.* Even when *access* is improved, studies indicate that different groups effectively *use* health care services unequally. The introduction of Medicare to the elderly, for example, had the effect of providing more use by the relatively wealthy than by the poor and by whites than by members of other races. While variation in use is likely to occur in any system, efforts should be made to reduce disparities in use on the basis of income and race.

(c) *Wide range of service.* Primary care must deal with a multiplicity and variety of needs which spread beyond narrow medical needs. A successful primary care system will reach out actively to the population it serves, and will deal, together with other social institutions, with nonmedical factors affecting health.

(d) *High quality of medical care.* American medicine prides itself on the high level of its scientific and technological development. Its accomplishments in many areas, particularly on the secondary and tertiary levels, have been spectacular. Yet the quality of care at the primary level varies considerably even when there is no difficulty of access. Standards must be maintained for physicians and for other health professionals, and quality controls improved and intensified. The effectiveness of care should be measured in terms of health maintenance as well as response to episodic illness and disability.

(e) *Continuity of service.* Effective primary health care will deal with each individual's problems in terms of his history, his family, his social and occupational background and the totality of his health care needs. As corollary, the patient should be cared for by a variety of specialized personnel when necessary, but in a systematic, coordinated way. Information about each patient should also be maintained in a systematic way, and methods developed for rapid transfer of such information.

(f) *Coordination of institutions.* The primary care system serves as a coordinating force for the consumer. In addition, it must provide appropriate staff affiliations for the primary care providers at nearby hospitals and access to social service agencies. Of special importance is the provisions of hospital staff affiliations for all practicing physicians desiring them.

(g) *Educative responsibilities.* The primary care system should perform an educative function on a one-to-one basis and also by sponsoring group activities and even by utilizing the media to reach larger groups.

(h) *Human support services.* Human support functions, which traditionally were provided by family and neighbors, such as care for the aged and assistance in times of family crises, must be recognized as an important adjunct to the primary care system.

(i) *Consumer participation.* The health care system has long been controlled almost entirely by the provider, primarily the physician. While systems of control will vary, it is important that the voice of consumers be heard to help guide the development and operations of primary care institutions. The consumer by himself and through representatives should have an impact on different levels—from greater responsiveness to specific complaints to participation in policy formulation and administrative organization.

12. A number of different types of organizations currently deliver primary care. Their contributions, strengths and weaknesses must be evaluated not only in terms of the present delivery of care but also as models for the future:

(a) The *private physician,* practicing alone or in privately-organized fee-for-service group practice, will remain the basis of primary care for many years. Because of his personal relationship with his patient and his assumption of responsibility for continuous service, the value of the service he provides should not be underrated. However, the solo practitioner is increasingly limited in terms of the breadth of services he can perform, and if his number continues to decrease, the burdens will grow too great for him to handle efficiently and adequately. Among the responses to this problem has been the development of multi- or single-specialty group practice and private clinics. These organizations often have certain advantages over solo practice, such as greater availability and arrangements for night service, and might become the base for more highly developed organizations utilizing other health professionals. However, there is no significant evidence to date that private group practice will effectively deliver the full range of primary care to a major part of the population.

(b) *Hospital outpatient departments,* while serving a large number of patients and possessing expertise and ready access to secondary facilities, have difficulty providing continuous service to a defined population group. These clinics are usually impersonal and fragmented in their approach and, as less prestigious appendages to hospitals, are unlikely in their present form to provide a strong model for the organization of a primary care system. However, a great deal of effective primary care is presently being provided through outpatient clinics, and until other methods of delivery are developed these clinics will be an indispensable source of primary care in many communities.

(c) The *emergency room* of the hospital has become a primary care provider by default. While it serves the functions of entry and diagnosis for a specific complaint, it is not organized to provide continuous and coordinated primary health care.

(d) Without suggesting that it is the only model available, *prepaid group practice,* with emphasis on comprehensive care on a continuous basis, provides a much more promising model of integrating primary health care into a full program of health service. The high start-up cost of prepaid group practice and public unfamiliarity with this approach, and the fact that under some such plans there is a feeling that service tends to be impersonal, have caused the relatively slow growth of prepaid group practice, and at present less than 4 percent of primary care is provided by such organizations.

(e) Recently developed *neighborhood health centers* and similar groups offer substantial potential for meeting the criteria for the delivery of a full primary care package, primarily in the breadth of service and involvement of the community. However, as currently constituted, the neighborhood health centers suffer from certain defects. They serve only a highly restricted population, their cost per unit of service appears high and they have not successfully integrated primary care with other levels of health services.

It is essential to recognize in considering the effectiveness of the above and other forms of primary care organizations that none of them is likely to achieve its objective in isolation, but must be effectively related to secondary and tertiary care providers.

13. Our experience to date leads to the conclusion that there is no one model of a primary health care organization that has demonstrated its superiority and validity to the extent that it should be fostered at the expense of other approaches. Rather, the public interest would be best served by encouraging the various institutions and approaches described above, and the development of others, so long as they meet basic standards of service. Reimbursement methods should not discriminate against any of the various models, with the caveat that a minimum cluster of primary care service be offered by those providers receiving governmental reimbursement. At the same time, the federal government should be prepared to provide funds for capital needs and special services to encourage the development and operation of new institutions and arrangements where financial and institutional barriers exist. Consumers should be given an opportunity for choice among primary care

providers and given with the information needed to make rational choices.

14. The more than 6,000 community hospitals in the United States have come to play a significant primary care role, largely as a catch-all for the shortcomings of the entire system. This is a role that hospitals are not presently designed to fill, and this growing burden is often seen as interfering with the traditional secondary care responsibilities of hospitals. There is an inherent conflict within the hospital structure between the hospital's main interest in providing secondary care, and its subsidiary involvement in maintaining primary care services, usually through an outpatient clinic. However, it must be recognized that because other delivery methods have often been inadequate, hospitals in many communities have assumed an indispensable role in offering primary care, primarily through outpatient clinics. Hospitals have the advantage of being firmly established in most communities, including inner-city areas, and having a pool of skilled manpower and access to financial resources. In the long run, adequate primary health services can be provided under the auspices of hospitals only with changes in the way they are presently controlled and operated. Where primary care units are formed in connection with an established hospital, these primary health care units should be created with a degree of self-identity and bargaining autonomy.

15. One of the concomitants of the emerging structure of the primary care delivery system has been the development of new health practitioners. The physician has now been supplemented by physician extenders such as the physician's assistant, the MEDEX and the nurse practitioner. The private physician has in many cases built up a support team to permit him to serve a larger number of patients and to add to the breadth and sophistication of the service he provides. Also, neighborhood family health workers in many neighborhood health centers have made a major contribution by performing limited but valuable functions. The development of new types of health manpower is a welcome sign and should be encouraged. Preliminary indications are that they are performing and will perform a valuable function. In spite of the optimism shared by the members of the Forum, certain questions remain unanswered with respect to these new professionals:

(a) It is not at all clear that they will lead to a reduction in the cost of service. Their contributions to date appear to be more in the area of improving access and strengthening the scope and quality of service rather than lowering costs.

(b) Primary medical care is moving increasingly to more organized delivery methods. The introduction of a "team approach" has, however, led in many cases to administrative difficulties and even to conflict among the providers. Experiments with different patterns of team organizations should be encouraged.

(c) The introduction of more nonphysicians into the health care process raises additional problems of evaluating and controlling a quality of service, which is already a problem. Moreover, in developing standards for evaluation, there is a danger that the introduction of a certification process will rigidify these new professional groups and prevent the flexibility and innovation that is so badly needed. At this stage, overlapping functions are to be preferred to a structure of a clearly defined division of responsibilities.

(d) It might be thought that consumers would not readily accept nonphysicians as health care providers, but the limited experience to date has indicated instead widespread acceptance and even enthusiasm.

16. Recruitment to the medical profession and the nature of medical education have an important influence on attitudes, values and goals in the medical profession. In the last few decades medical education has been dominated and controlled by the medical specialists; high status, as well as financial rewards, has gone to the student who made a career in a narrow specialty. While this type of education has led to great scientific advances and American preeminence at the secondary and tertiary levels of health care, it has also had the effect of downgrading the aspirations of medical students who seek to enter the primary care area. If primary care is to improve, it must become a highly respected aspect of the medical profession; indeed, the skills and knowledge required of the competent primary physician are more extensive than those of the specialist.

17. There are some positive signs that the medical education is changing to meet the challenge of primary care.

(a) Students in the past few years have appeared to be more interested in practice in the primary care area.

(b) A new certified specialty in family medicine has been established in the past three years and the number of residencies training for the specialty has increased markedly since 1970. Development of this specialty should be encouraged. Flexible new experimental educational formats should be developed for family medicine, general internal medicine and pediatrics. In particular, family medicine curricula should be broadened to include more content in community-related health problems.

Despite some encouraging signs, America's medical education is still dominated by a bias toward specialty medicine which should be offset by new, vigorous attention to primary care. Government grants and financial incentives should be used to promote primary care education in the medical training institutions, just as in an earlier period large-scale governmental support for scientific research influenced these institutions to orient themselves more strongly toward science and research.

18. A very real problem exists in financing graduate medical education in primary care specialties where much of the training is obtained in the ambulatory environment. Hospital based specialty training is currently financed through third party reimbursement for hospital services. No analogous mechanism is available for the financing of ambulatory training, even if funding

for ambulatory services were adequate. The problem is accentuated in community settings where no formal relationship to a hospital exists. Some new means to pay for this vital aspect of training must be found.

19. At present, physicians, nurses, and physician assistants are typically trained entirely separately. Experience indicates that this separate training makes it extremely difficult for them to work together later in primary health care teams; additional difficulties are created by sex stereotypes in the medical professions which tend adversely to affect working relationships among health professionals. While a common curriculum or educational system is not necessary, there should be more joint training, and such joint training should commence at the very beginning of the professional schooling.

III. The Financing of Primary Care

20. Our methods of financing health care in the past and at present profoundly affect the type of care that is provided. In the past, insurance systems—both private and governmental—and methods of public support for health care have focused primarily on major illnesses and disabilities requiring hospitalization. Third-party payment for hospitalization has had the effect of strengthening secondary and tertiary care, at the expense of primary care.

21. The future financing of the health care system will undoubtedly accelerate the reliance on third party payments, through which the provider is paid by governmental or private insurance programs or by public or private subsidies. Already approximately 90 percent of hospital care and 60 percent of physician services are paid for in this way. It can be expected that there will be a major national health insurance program within the next few years. That funding system, when it comes, should not only finance the health care system but should play a direct role in ensuring that the present delivery system is reshaped to provide, among other important things, an adequate level of primary care available to all.

22. The principal elements of a satisfactory financing system should be:

(a) *Universality of insurance system.* A national health insurance program should be available to all—both for reasons of equity and public acceptability.

(b) *Equitable effect of insurance system.* Some symposium participants believe that even with equal financial access and special supplemental support, the poor and minority groups will receive less than an equitable share of health care. They believe that the financing method should, therefore, provide larger financial benefits to the poor than to the more wealthy. One means of doing this would be the establishment of deductible and coinsurance features scaled with income, subject to a maximum limit. Other symposium participants believe that a universal insurance system, with equal financial access for all, accompanied by supplemental measures for the disadvantaged groups, would provide an equitable system, and further that graduated deductibles and coinsurance would create problems of administration and equality.

(c) *The goal of comprehensive and continuance maintenance of the population's health.* An important part of a health maintenance system must be an emphasis on preventive medicine, that is, concern not only for treating a specific illness but also for preventing further health problems through periodic evaluation, immunization, counseling, education and the like.

(d) *Coverage of all major areas of personal health care.* It would be unwise, for example, to establish a government-organized insurance program covering only "catastrophic" illness and disability.

(e) *Influence on costs.* A new health insurance system must provide mechanisms to inhibit insofar as possible cost inflation through incentives, disincentives and limitations on payments services.

(f) *Quality standards.* It is not possible to deal effectively with costs without dealing also with the quality of services rendered: reimbursement mechanisms which emphasize the efficient delivery of health care should not encourage the delivery of inferior care. The development of measurable standards for service is an extremely difficult task, but it must be undertaken on a high priority basis with the participation of the medical profession, other health professionals as well as consumers of health services. These standards should not be limited to medical services, but should provide a basis for evaluation of the provision of the broader components of primary care.

(g) *Effect on delivery methods.* The financing system should maintain strict neutrality as to methods and forms of institutions delivering health care, including primary care, although, of course, standards of quality and scope of care must be established. One of the best, although by no means perfect, methods to promote a responsive, humane, and effective health care system and to avoid bureaucratic domination is to encourage diversity among different types of delivery.

23. No system of health insurance or care delivery will solve all the problems of access and usage of medical care by disadvantaged population groups. In large measure, inadequacy of medical services for blacks and other disadvantaged minorities is not a fully isolatable problem but rather a manifestation of deep-rooted interrelated problems of underemployment, inferior education, cultural alienation and a generally deprived social and physical environment. The inadequacy of health care in rural areas is related to pervasive economic and sociological issues. For this reason there must be emphasis on increased programs and institutions directed primarily at solving these problems, even before a national health insurance system is enacted. However, in acting to meet specific and immediate needs of particular groups, it is important that these be consistent with a long-run strategy to improve primary

care on a nationwide basis.

24. The needs of primary health care must be viewed as a part of the total health care system; and in turn, the needs of the health care system as a whole must be seen in the context of the multiplicity of social needs in the United States today. In assessing priorities, the development of improved primary care should be seen as the most important need in the health care system. Those with the responsibility to allocate resources in the area of health care should place continued and increased emphasis on access to primary care by disadvantaged groups—inner-city residents, racial and linguistic minorities, the rural population, the aged and the poor and working poor. In that effort, the providers of health services must be enlisted as willing cooperators. This is particularly true in primary health care—where so large a component of the service required by the patient is humane concern, psychological support and the personal touch.

MATTHEW NIMETZ, ESQ.
Rapporteur

V APPENDIX

THE SUN VALLEY FORUM ON NATIONAL HEALTH, INC.

The Sun Valley Forum on National Health is a nonprofit educational organization incorporated in 1970 under the laws of Idaho. The purpose of the Forum is to work toward the improvement of the health of Americans and of the health care delivery system. The Forum seeks this objective through educational activities—the sponsorship of symposia, conferences and lectures and the preparation and publication of books, papers and reports. Governed by a board of directors of medical professionals and lay leaders, the Forum endeavors to carry out its programs at the highest possible level of quality and excellence.

Activities of the Forum center in Sun Valley, a facility well suited and equipped for sustained serious discussion. The Forum's symposia bring together leaders and experts to meet, to share ideas, and to review expert papers on aspects of the nation's health problems. Symposium participants include professionals in all health related fields as well as other persons associated with or interested in health affairs, such as representatives of consumers, businessmen, public officials and educators.

Since its founding in 1970 the Forum has held three such symposia. These were major undertakings, each lasting six days, involving about 30 participants, concentrating on a group of specially commissioned working papers, and each producing a final report of the symposium.

Activities of the Sun Valley Forum on National Health are supported by grants from individuals, corporations, foundations and the Department of Health, Education and Welfare's National Center for Health Services Research and Development.

The views presented in this book are those of the authors and symposium participants and not necessarily those of the officers, directors, or staff members of The Sun Valley Forum on National Health, Inc.

FORUM OFFICERS

Chairman
Bayless Manning
President of the Council
    on Foreign Relations
New York, New York

Executive Director
Robert G. Lindee
Vice President
The Henry J. Kaiser Family Foundation
Palo Alto, California

Secretary
David Lincoln
Elam, Burke, Jeppesen, Evans
    and Boyd, Attorneys at Law
Sun Valley, Idaho

Treasurer
James E. Phelps
Vice President
First Security Bank of Idaho
Boise, Idaho

BOARD OF DIRECTORS

Howard R. Bowen
Chancellor
Claremont University Center
Claremont, California

William C. Janss
Sun Valley Company
Sun Valley, Idaho

Philip R. Lee, M.D.
Director
Health Policy Program
University of California
San Francisco, California

John B. Fery
President and Chief Executive Officer
Boise Cascade Corporation
Boise, Idaho

Melvin A. Glasser
Director of Social Security
United Automobile Workers Union
Detroit, Michigan

Margaret Mahoney
Vice President
The Robert Wood Johnson Foundation
Princeton, New Jersey

Richard Goodwin
President
The Johns-Manville Corporation
Denver, Colorado

Robert B. Miller, Jr.
Publisher
The Idaho Statesman
Boise, Idaho

The Hon. Averell Harriman
Washington, D.C.

Franklin D. Murphy
Chairman of the Board
Times-Mirror Company
Los Angeles, California

John Hogness, M.D.
President, Institute of Medicine
Washington, D.C.

Gerard Piel
President
Scientific American
New York, New York

Charles Schultze
Senior Policy Fellow
The Brookings Institution
Washington, D.C.

Mitchell W. Spellman, M.D.
Dean
Charles R. Drew
Postgraduate Medical School
Los Angeles, California

INDEX